How Do I Do This
When I Can't See What I'm Doing?

Information Processing for the Visually Disabled

Gerald Jahoda

**National Library Service
for the Blind and
Physically Handicapped**

The Library of Congress

Washington 1993

For sale by the U.S. Government Printing Office
Superintendent of Documents, Mail Stop: SSOP, Washington, DC 20402-9328
ISBN 0-16-041749-X

Library of Congress Cataloging-in-Publication Data

Jahoda, Gerald, 1925–
    How do I do this when I can't see what I'm doing : information
processing for the visually disabled / Gerald Jahoda.
        p.   cm.
    Includes bibliographical references and index.
    ISBN 0-8444-0785-2 (pbk.)
    1. Visually handicapped — United States — Life skills guides.
2. Blind — United States — Life skills guides.   I. Title.
HV1795.J34   1993   93-986
362.4'1—dc20   CIP

To Pat, my wife, my friend,
and my sighted companion,
par excellence.

Contents

Preface

This book is written for persons who have a visual disability and who wish to learn about alternate ways of processing information, including reading, writing, and organizing notes, as well as doing other everyday tasks. While loss of sight is debilitating and devastating when it first strikes, it need not remain so. Techniques and devices are available today that enable visually impaired persons to walk on their own, to read and write, and to perform other daily tasks independently. Much of this book is devoted to describing ways for visually impaired persons to process information so that they can become independent.

The first person plural "we" used in the book refers to the fact that the author is also visually impaired and has, therefore, used most of the techniques and devices described. I have lost most of my sight due to retinitis pigmentosa, a genetic eye disease that destroys the pigments in the retina. When my sight deteriorated so that I could no longer read print, type, or walk without bumping into things, I feared that I had come to the end of my world. But slowly, very slowly, I learned the various skills that now enable me to do most of the things that I did before.

All of us who face loss of sight have to go through this period of adjustment and transition. It may take a year or it may take longer, depending on how good we are at solving problems. We can and should draw on outside help to shorten this period of adjustment. Rehabilitation teachers can teach us useful skills. Other visually disabled persons can tell us how they overcame problems that we now face. It is important to keep in mind that thousands upon thousands of visually impaired persons have made a successful adjustment to their disability and are living active, productive, and enjoyable lives.

The first chapter of the book describes ways in which we can adjust to loss of sight. The second chapter deals with the use of computers by visually disabled persons. The basics of computer operations, adaptive computer input and output devices, and commonly used application programs are described. In chapter 3, I discuss personal information management systems—the ways we seek information and the ways we organize and store information for future use. Chapter 4 lists types of jobs held by visually disabled persons and reviews steps that we can take to enter or reenter the job market. Leisure activities are discussed in chapter 5. These activities are grouped into three categories: those requiring physical effort, those that emphasize mental effort, and volunteer activities. The last chapter is on the blindness system—organizations of and for visually disabled persons. Benefits provided by these and other organizations are discussed.

A comment is in order about why reading is discussed in both the chapter on personal information management and the chapter on leisure activities. When we read for school or work, we typically do so for a specific purpose—to gather information for a report, to prepare for an assignment, or to look up a fact that will help us in decision making. With such reading, we usually perform related tasks: we take notes and we organize these notes for subsequent use, hence the discussion of this type of reading with other information management tasks. Reading for recreation, on the other hand, is typically not done for a specific purpose; it is a way to spend leisure time enjoyably. This type of reading is discussed along with other leisure activities in the chapter devoted to such activities.

The text of each chapter is followed by a list of references and resources, including books and magazine articles covering the issues discussed. When they are available, recorded books are referenced. Also listed under resources are some government and private organizations that provide services to visually disabled persons.

Acknowledgments

I would like to acknowledge the help of Ellen Griswald and Beth Logan in reading aloud and editing the manuscript.

My thanks go to my wife, Pat Jahoda, not only for helping me with various tasks associated with writing but for her unfailing support and encouragement.

Tallahassee, Florida
July 1992

1. Everyday living skills

Before we can adjust to our loss of sight, we have to accept it as a fact of life. When we can look at our situation objectively, we realize that we can still do most of the things we have done before, although we will have to do some things differently. The fact that you are reading this book indicates that you are well on the way to accepting your disability; adjusting is the next step. The techniques and devices described in this chapter have been developed over the years by blind persons and by sighted persons working with blind persons. Thanks to their efforts, blind persons are now able to do most things for themselves and to enjoy normal lives. Some of the techniques and devices mentioned here are more fully described in the resource guide *Living with Low Vision* and in the other books listed and briefly described at the end of this chapter.

The devices and supplies mentioned here are available from mail-order houses that specialize in products for the blind. The names, addresses, and toll-free telephone numbers of some of these companies are also listed at the end of the chapter.

The home

A house or apartment becomes a home when we feel comfortable living in it. Three elements that contribute to being comfortable are lighting, color scheme, and arrangement of furniture.

The type of lighting that is best for us depends on our particular eye disease; lighting that is too bright for one person may not be bright enough for another. Trial and error is a good way to find the optimum lighting. We can choose the type of light bulb (fluorescent or incandescent), the strength of the bulb, and its placement in a room. Fluorescent light does not cast shadows and produces less glare than incandescent light. It does not have to be mounted in rectangular fixtures (which fit better in an institution than in a home); round fluorescent bulbs that fit into regular sockets can be purchased. Also available are special incandescent light bulbs that produce less glare than the regular ones. We may want fluorescent lights in places where more light is needed: the bathroom, the kitchen, and the study. In the bathroom, we may be able to see ourselves better with an illuminated magnifying mirror. Special light fixtures and light bulbs are available from mail-order houses. Floor lamps might be replaced with ceiling lamps to reduce glare and provide more open space in a room. Curtains or blinds are effective to shield us from direct sunlight.

How well we can see our surroundings also depends on the color of the walls, the ceilings, and the carpets as well as on the contrast between furniture and background color. Light colors, such as white, beige, or tan, are suggested for walls, ceilings, and carpets. Darker colors on furniture, light switchplates, and electrical outlets make them easier to see.

Furniture should be kept in one place to avoid painful surprises. Doors should be either open or shut—never partly open—so that we do not hurt ourselves. For a fuller discussion of these matters on a room-by-room basis, see *Making Life More Livable* by Irving R. Dickman, listed in the references.

Tasks of everyday living

As sighted persons, we performed most everyday tasks—such as turning off the alarm clock, selecting wardrobe for the day, or pouring a cup of coffee—without giving them much thought. Some of these tasks—for example, turning off the alarm clock—can still be done in the same way and without thinking about them; other tasks—such as selecting what clothes to wear or pouring a cup of coffee—must be done differently. In general, the difference in doing a task now is to supplement or substitute touch, hearing, and sometimes smell for sight.

Tasks that we do every day typically consist of two basic steps performed one or more times. The first step is to locate something; the second step is to do something with what we have located. The steps of locating and performing an action are repeated until the task is completed. For example, to heat a dish in the microwave oven, we locate the dish in the refrigerator by shape or memory and pull it out. Then we place the dish in the microwave oven. We locate the numeric key pad and key in the number of seconds that we want the dish to be heated, locate the heating option buttons and push the appropriate one, then locate and push the "on" button.

Locating an item

Some items we locate because we know that they are there, such as the button that shuts off the clock radio alarm. We remember that the radio is on top of the nightstand and the alarm shut-off button is in the upper right-hand corner of the radio.

Locating items by physical characteristics

Some items can be selected from among similar items by their size, shape, or other physical characteristics. We may be able to identify a key on the keychain by feeling for its size and shape. We can use this technique for identifying coins too. Our coins differ in size and in having smooth or serrated edges, so they can be recognized by a combination of these features. Pennies are small and have smooth edges, nickels are large and have smooth edges, dimes are small and have serrated edges, and quarters are large and have serrated edges.

In some countries, paper money of different denominations differs in size and can be recognized that way. We cannot recognize dollar bills by size, but we can differentiate a five-dollar from a ten-dollar bill by folding the two bills differently in our billfold. A five-dollar bill might be folded in half lengthwise while a ten-dollar bill might be folded in half sideways. Twenty-dollar bills might have a corner folded and one-dollar bills might be placed in the billfold unfolded. This is an inexpensive way to differentiate bills if we do it right. I remember giving a hot dog vendor what I thought was a five-dollar bill and telling him to keep the change.

His effusive thanks suggested that I might have given him a bill of a larger denomination. The bill folding technique does not give a clue about the denomination of a bill that is given to us. There are electronic devices that will tell us this or we can just ask the person who gives us the bill.

Marking items

If the item that we seek does not have a physical characteristic that enables us to differentiate it from similar items, we can give it such a characteristic. Since the objective of marking an item is to distinguish it from similar items, we have to consider first what aspect of the item to use for making this distinction. For shirts, it could be the color, length of sleeve, or type of collar. The length of the sleeve and the type of collar can be determined by touch. The color of the shirt cannot be sensed by touch, and, since color is an important selection criterion, we will use it for our example.

What colors should we identify? That depends on two factors: the colors of the shirts that we own and the selection criteria that we want to use. Let's say we want to mark our shirts so that we select an appropriate color for the blue suit that we want to wear. We can mark the shirts by their colors—say, white, blue, red, green, or gray—and pick a color that goes with a blue suit. Or we can mark the shirts by the color of the suit with which they can be worn. This entails developing a color scheme based on the suits that we have—say, blue, grey, and brown—and marking the suits as well as the shirts with these colors. Once this color scheme is developed, ties and socks can be similarly marked.

We have chosen the colors to code for each item of clothing— namely, blue, gray, and brown. The second choice is what, if any, abbreviation to use for each color. We could use the word "blue," but an abbreviation is preferable because it is faster to read and takes less space on the tag or the garment. The abbreviation "bl" rather than the letter "b" is suggested, since the letter "b" can stand for either blue or brown. In this example, the abbreviations for colors are "bl," "br," and "gy." (The letter "g" could be used, but this letter could also be used for the color green, and one never knows when green suits might become fashionable.) The three colors can also be symbolized by numbers—say, 1, 2, and 3—

or by geometric shapes—such as circles, squares, and triangles. If a shirt, tie, or pair of socks goes with more than one color suit, all applicable colors are marked. Women's apparel can be similarly marked. Jewelry that goes with a particular color scheme can be placed in marked bags.

There is one more decision that needs to be made: how do we physically mark the item? We can either put the mark on the item itself or place a tag on it. For those of us with some sight, a mark with a thick waterproof pen works. For those without any sight, the mark must be in raised letters, raised numbers, or geometric designs. The letters or numbers can be regular print or braille; if we use braille, we need only remember numbers and letters of the alphabet. Braille marking devices are available from mail-order houses. For some items, marking with a single raised dot is best. Such dots on adhesive backing are available from mail-order houses or can be produced at home with nail polish.

Another option to consider when marking with phrases of two or more words is a system that uses a special tape recorder that can record on and read strips of magnetic tape attached to cards or tags. The recorder is called Voxcom® and the system is described in *Seeing with the Brain*, a book by Mildred Frank cited in the references. A strip of magnetic tape is attached to a tag, which is then inserted in the tape recorder. The words or phrases are recorded on the tape. To play the words or phrases, the tag with recorded tape is inserted into the specially designed tape recorder.

The mental map

A mental map is an image that gives us the location of various items in relation to a reference point. Let us take as an example the numeric keypad on a touchtone telephone, some microwave ovens, or a computer keyboard. We view the numeric keypad as four rows of three keys. Our reference point is the 5 key, which we can mark with a raised dot. Once we get to this key (and assuming we know that the 9 key is on the third row) we can locate any key on the keypad.

All of us have a mental map or image of the face of a clock as a set of numbers within a circle. Looking down on the circle, the number 12 is on top, the number 3 is ninety degrees to the right, the number 6 is another ninety degrees to the right, and the number 9 still another ninety degrees to the right and ninety degrees from the number 12, making this a circle of 360 degrees. If we think of a dinner plate as a clock, we can be told where different foods have been placed on the plate. For example, the meat is from 12 to 4, the potatoes are from 4 to 7, broccoli is from 7 to 9, and parsley is at 11. This mapping technique can also be used to indicate the location of items near the plate. For example, the water glass is above 1 and the wine glass is at 3. This technique is very helpful not only to locate food we want to eat but also to avoid accidental consumption of parsley, lemon slices, and other items placed there for decoration.

Carrying out the task

Locating an item is usually the preliminary step to doing something with it. We carry out some of these tasks by supplementing or substituting touch or hearing for sight.

Using the sense of touch

Here is an example of substituting touch for sight. Liquid can be poured into a glass to a desired level by using a method described by Ralph Read (see references). We hold the glass in one hand, with the index finger inside the glass. The tip of the index finger is at the desired liquid level. We hold the bottle in the other hand and pour the liquid into the glass until it touches the index finger.

Margaret Smith (see references) makes a simple suggestion for directing toothpaste onto the toothbrush, a suggestion that would have spared me much frustration over the years. One squeezes the toothpaste onto a finger and then transfers the toothpaste to the toothbrush.

Using the sense of hearing

Devices are available that provide information by beeps, clicks, or spoken message. One electronic device emits a single beep when a five-dollar bill is inserted into it, two beeps when a ten-dollar bill is inserted, and three beeps when a twenty-dollar bill is inserted. A one-dollar bill causes no beeps. This device costs several hundred dollars and is useful for people who use a cash register.

Thermostats that make an audible click for every unit of change in the temperature setting are available. To change the temperature setting we place the pointer on a temperature marked with a raised dot and move it the required number of clicks to the left or right.

Battery-operated talking watches and clocks are another example of devices used by hearing rather than seeing. We press a button to hear the time. We press another button to set the time or the alarm and are given the changes in settings, hour by hour and minute by minute, audibly.

We can now weigh ourselves in private with a battery-operated talking bathroom scale. We weigh ourselves on such a scale by pushing a button that invites us to step on the scale. After a couple of seconds of standing on the scale, our weight is read out. We are then told either "good-bye" or "have a nice day." We can get our weight in pounds or kilos, and we can be told if we have lost or gained weight since the last weighing. The scale will also tell us by voice when its battery is low.

A talking thermometer tells us our body temperature and a talking kitchen scale tells us the weight of ingredients. An audible device, called a liquid-level indicator, helps us pour liquid into a container if we prefer not to stick our finger into it. It is battery-operated, attaches to the container into which the liquid is to be poured, and emits a sound when the liquid reaches the desired level.

Getting around

Persons with limited or no sight can get from place to place on foot using a sighted guide, a white cane, or a dog guide.

Using a sighted guide

The sighted guide or sighted companion technique is the simplest of the three techniques to learn because it is the most intuitive, the most natural. We walk next to but a half step behind the sighted companion, except when crowded conditions require walking single file. We hold the companion's right arm just above the elbow with the left hand if we are left-handed or the companion's left arm with our right hand if we are right-handed. As we walk, we will follow the body motion of the companion. He or she will stop at street crossings, steps, and other deviations from a level path and will tell us if a step is up or down, if a door opens from the left or the right, and whether it must be pushed or pulled. In crowds and tight passages, such as in restaurants, the sighted companion will indicate by movement of arm that we should switch hands and walk behind him or her, single file. When we are guided to a car, the guide will place our hand at the top of the opened car door or the back of the seat so we can tell which way the seat is facing. Because of the simplicity of the technique, guiding can be taught to sighted persons who have only casual contact with us, such as waiters, cab drivers, and hairdressers.

Using a white cane

The white cane is a symbol that tends to mean one thing to an observer and quite another to its user. To the sighted person, the cane often means that the user is an object of sympathy, someone who needs help. To its user, the cane represents the ability to move from place to place at any time and without outside help. As newly blinded persons our perception of a white cane may be the same as a sighted person's and this may explain in part our reluctance to use this tool. This, at least, was my experience. For a long time I would not even consider it, despite many incidents caused by lack of vision. I barked my shins on fire hydrants, hit my head on stop signs, and broke my nose on a telephone pole. People attributed my behavior to a problem with alcohol or drugs and suggested that I lay off the stuff. It was only when I narrowly escaped being run over by a car that I decided to carry a white cane. I use the term "carry" advisedly, because I planned to use the cane to warn people of my vision problem and not for its intended purpose as a mobility aid. The difference in people's attitudes toward me with and without a white cane was quite remarkable. Without a cane, people disapproved of me and told me so. With a cane, people offer help, even when I do not need it.

There finally came a time when I thought it would be a good idea to learn how to use the white cane in the way that it is intended to be used. A phone call to the local agency serving blind persons brought forth an orientation and mobility instructor, a professional trained to teach the use of the white cane as well as other mobility and everyday living skills. Orientation and mobility instructors still make house calls, since their job is to help us cope in our surroundings.

8

When the instructor first came to my house, we discussed and agreed on the objectives of my instruction. My objectives were to be able to walk on my own around the neighborhood, both for exercise and to buy things at the local store. My instructor prepared a tactile map of the neighborhood, made with braille dots. Then my mobility training began.

The first thing I had to learn was to walk a straight line, a skill that I seemed to have forgotten over the years. When I was able to perform this task, I learned how to hold the white cane, with arm extended, in the left hand if we are left-handed and in the right hand if we are right-handed. As an extension of the hand, the cane enables us to follow a given path, and to sense and therefore avoid obstacles on that path. As we walk, we sweep the cane from side to side and tap it on both sides. The sweeping motion is to sense obstacles in front of us. The angle of the sweep should be wide enough to protect the body from shoulder to shoulder against obstacles in our way. Tapping to the left and the right serves two purposes. It enables us to follow the path by sensing for the "shore-line"—the line between pavement and grass or other differentiating composition. Tapping also serves to alert us to curbs, steps, or other obstacles on the ground.

The feel, sounds, and smells of the area in which I walk provide me with useful clues. The sounds of cars on a busy street a few blocks away tell me that I am walking in a particular direction. The barking of a dog used to tell me I was passing a particular house near a street corner, but the dog has gotten used to me now and no longer barks. Another temporary landmark is the smell of a bank of honeysuckle vines in the spring. The year-round smell of a pizza parlor is another directional clue. Fire hydrants, stop signs, and telephone poles are no longer objects to bump into but have become landmarks useful for finding my way.

Using a dog guide

The third method of travelling on foot is with the aid of a dog guide. If we want a dog guide, we must go to dog guide school and stay there for about four weeks. The school will match us with a dog that has already undergone some training. It is important that we get along with the dog and that the dog gets along with us, since the two of us will spend a lot of time together. In fact, the dog will be our constant companion for a number of years. During our days at the school, we will learn to walk with our dog to specific destinations, board buses, and go into stores and restaurants. We will learn that our dog guide does not know where we are going, that we will have to instruct him to go straight, left, or right. The dog will stop at a street crossing and will not cross the street until it is safe to do so. Our part of the bargain is to groom, feed, exercise, and, in general, keep the dog in good health and spirits. This includes praising him when he is doing his job. Andrew Potock has written an amusing and informative article about one man's experience with a dog guide (see references).

Going to a restaurant

No matter who cooks at home or how good this cook is, most of us like to eat out occasionally, if not often, and limited sight should not deprive us of this pleasure. Here are pointers intended to make eating out fun. In addition to requesting a smoking or nonsmoking area, we might want to ask for a table with lighting that is best for our eyes. The sighted companion or waiter guiding us to the table should be asked to place our hand on the back of our chair. Ask the companion or waiter to read the menu aloud. If it is a long menu (such as those typical of Chinese restaurants) we might speed up the process by specifying seafood, chicken, meat, or vegetables as a main dish. We tell the waiter about our visual problem and what help we need. If we order a salad, we might ask to have it served on a large plate so we can cut lettuce and other salad ingredients without having part of the salad spill off the plate. We also ask the waiter to tell us when he fills our glass with wine or water; it is disconcerting to drink from a glass that we thought was almost empty but that turns out to be full. We could figure this out from the weight of the glass, but we do not always think about this.

When the main course arrives, we ask for the location of different items on the plate by means of the face-of-the-clock method. Consider the European method of eating, not because of its snob value but because of its utility. The Europeans hold forks in the left hand and knives in the right hand. The knife is not only used for cutting but also for guiding food onto the fork—very handy when we have peas or other small items to put on the fork. Eating chicken with our fingers and using them to help in other ways are acceptable.

When it comes time to settle the accounts, we can ask our companion or the waiter for the amount due. The methods for identifying money, discussed earlier in this chapter, will be helpful for leaving a tip and paying the bill. Some blind persons and a lot of sighted ones prefer to pay with a credit card. Both the bill and the tip can be charged with the card.

The main thing about eating out is to be relaxed about the whole thing and to enjoy it. We have all made social faux pas and survived them. In fact, some of these faux pas make very fine stories that we can tell on ourselves.

This chapter has dealt with everyday living skills, sometimes called independent living skills. These are skills that all newly blinded persons need to learn, and we can learn them with the aid of rehabilitation teachers. Instructions in independent living skills are provided free of charge by state agencies for the blind. These agencies are discussed in the chapter on jobs, since they play an important role not only in helping us to adjust to loss of sight but also in helping us keep the job we now have or find a new job.

References

Dickman, Irving R. *Making Life More Livable: Simple Adaptations for the Homes of Blind and Visually Impaired Older People.* New York: American Foundation for the Blind, 1983. (RC 22319)[*]

This book has many good suggestions for making each room in the home more livable for visually impaired persons. The question-and-answer technique is used to discuss lights, colors, marking items to be sensed, and other topics.

---

[*]Books with an RC number are recorded on cassette by the National Library Service for the Blind and Physically Handicapped (NLS). The books can be borrowed from NLS regional libraries. Details of this service are given in chapter 5.

Frank, Mildred. *Seeing with the Brain*, rev. ed. Indianapolis: Council of Citizens with Low Vision, 1991. (Available in large print or cassette from CCLVI, 5707 Brockton Drive, No. 302, Indianapolis, IN 46220.)

In twenty chapters, the author deals with a range of topics of concern to visually disabled persons, including mobility, labeling methods, shopping, color coding clothing, personal grooming, and filing recipes.

Living with Low Vision: A Resource Guide for People with Sight Loss. Lexington, KY: Resources for Rehabilitation, 1990.

This edition is in large print. In addition to chapters on reading, jobs, technology, adjustment, and recreation, there are chapters on self-help groups and services for children, adolescents, veterans, and people with both vision and hearing loss, as well as chapters on specific eye diseases. Relevant publications, including tapes, and names and addresses of organizations are listed in each chapter.

Potock, Andrew. "Dash and Me: An Intense Relationship Has Its Ups and Downs." *Life* 11(July 1988):73.

The author writes about life with Dash, his dog guide. Their training and subsequent experiences with each other are told with good humor.

Read, Ralph. *When the Cook Can't Look: A Cooking Handbook for the Blind and Visually Impaired.* The author, 1981. (RC 17940)

The recorded book is both tone-indexed and voice-indexed. Part One deals with techniques used in the kitchen, including opening containers, pouring, and measuring. Part Two provides recipes for breakfast, lunch, and dinner dishes. The appendix lists the recipes according to three levels of difficulty.

Smith, Margaret M. *If Blindness Strikes, Don't Strike Out: A Lively Look at Living with Visual Impairment.* Springfield, IL: Charles C Thomas, 1984. (RC 21060)

Good down-to-earth advice on a variety of topics of concern to visually disabled persons, including reading, personal recordkeeping, shopping, grooming, social graces, travelling, civil rights, and caring for children.

VISION Resource List. 13th ed. 1991. (Available from the VISION Foundation, Inc., 828 Mt. Auburn Street, Watertown, MA 02172.)

This is a list of 152 publications on topics such as cooking, recreation, and mobility aids. The list of resources as well as the listed publications are available from the VISION Foundation.

Younger, Vivian, and Jill Sardegna. *One Way or Another: A Guide to Independence for the Visually Impaired and Their Families*. San Jose: Sardegna Productions, 1991. (Available for eighteen dollars from Sardegna Productions, 710 Almondwood Way, San Jose, CA 95120.)

Includes chapters on rehabilitation programs, adaptive devices, daily living skills, handling paperwork, and changing family roles.

Resources—mail-order houses specializing in products for blind persons

American Foundation for the Blind
Products for People with Vision Problems
15 West 16th Street
New York, NY 10011
1-800-829-0500

Ann Morris Enterprises, Inc.
26 Horseshoe Lane
Levittown, NY 11756
1-516-292-9232

Bossert Specialties, Inc.
P.O. Box 15441
Phoenix, AZ 85060
1-800-776-5885

Independent Living Aids, Inc.
27 East Mall
Plainview, NY 11803
1-800-537-2118

Maxi Aids
42 Executive Boulevard
P.O. Box 3209
Farmingdale, NY 11735
1-800-522-6294

Science Products
P.O. Box 888
Southeastern, PA 19399
1-800-888-7400

The Store at the Massachusetts Association for the Blind
200 Ivy Street
Brookline, MA 02146
1-800-682-9200

Vis-Aids, Inc.
102-09 Jamaica Avenue
P.O. Box 26
Richmond Hill, NY 11418
1-800-346-9579

2. Computers as assistive devices

In 1986, IBM made a promotional offer that was hard to resist. The company offered college teachers a six-month loan of IBM personal computers with software, at no cost or obligation. At that time, I taught at Florida State University. Retinitis pigmentosa had prevented me from reading unmagnified print for about ten years. Print that I could read comfortably had to be in characters of about two-thirds of an inch high. I could read smaller print but had to make guesses on some words. My correspondence, lecture notes, and other writing had to be done by hand in large and bold lettering, as I could no longer use a typewriter. One of my colleagues had been encouraging me for about a year to use a computer, but the small characters on the computer monitor made me stick to handwriting with a thick pen. When I found out that the size of characters on the monitor could be doubled and that I could try it out for six months, I changed my mind and decided to use a computer.

And so, one fine day in May 1986, an IBM personal computer arrived in my office. It came packed in several boxes loaded on a dolly and wheeled in by a friendly IBM representative. When the boxes were unpacked and the equipment assembled, there sat on a table near my desk a brand new IBM personal computer, a monitor, a printer, a word processing program and other software, as well as pages and pages of instructions on how to use the computer and the software. If nothing else, the computer and the manuals were a nice addition to my office. Before the IBM representative departed, he started the computer, set it to the enlarged character mode, and wished me happy computing.

As I sat in front of the computer that day, I experienced the mixed emotions of elation and apprehension: elation because I could see how much more efficient the physical process of writing would become with a computer; apprehension because I have learned over the years that one gets nothing for nothing. Even though the equipment and software were free for the next six months, it would take time and effort before I could put the computer to use. My acquaintance with computers came from earlier days, before personal and user-friendly computers. It dated from a time when one brought a tray of punched cards to the computing center; a technician fed the cards into the card reader, the computer input device used at that time; then one waited at the computer center for a half-hour or longer until the program was run and the results were presented in the form of a printout. If the printout did not have the expected, needed, or desired information, the process was repeated as many times as necessary. On this day, there was no technician; instead, there was a monitor screen with a blinking signal saying, in effect, "It's your turn."

My first attempt was to write a letter on the computer. Even though this event happened more than six years ago, I remember it vividly. Writing a letter on the computer entails, as I found out later, calling up the word processing program, keying in the letter, correcting typos, naming the letter for filing, and printing and filing it. I could and did call up the word processing program but had no idea how to use it. Reading the program manuals would have been the thing to do, but I was too impatient for that; I wanted to learn by doing. I did, but it took a long time to prepare a very short letter. Not only did I not know the function of the function keys or other special keys, I did not know the location of any of the keys and I could not read the markings on the keys. Keying in the letter meant going back and forth from the keyboard to an enlarged illustration of it on my reading machine, which was located a few steps from the computer. When this laborious process was completed I printed the letter, but I did not save it because I didn't know how. Proofing the letter under the reading machine I found typos and had to key in the whole letter again. The second time I learned how to save it.

This and similar experiences taught me a few things. First, read the manual before beginning to use a new program. Second, read the manual whenever a problem appears. Third, have a computer buddy who can help you when you need it. Look for a person who does not make a neophyte feel stupid, can be interrupted, and does not give long lectures. Fourth, either memorize the location of all the keys on the keyboard or have an enlarged illustration of the keyboard at the computer. It helps to have raised dots on some frequently used keys, such as the delete and backspace keys.

When the six-month trial period was up, I was addicted to the computer and the university managed to let me keep it in the office. I now have a computer in my home office, on which this book was written.

An overview of computers

A computer is equipment or hardware that helps us perform a task. The task may be to type a letter, to arrange a list of names alphabetically, or to add the dollar amounts on the checks that we wrote last month. These and other tasks are done by a person and a computer in the same general way. Data, which are the words or numbers that the computer is to process, are fed to the computer by an input device. The input device is usually a keyboard similar to that on a typewriter. The computer processes the data it receives. Processing entails performing operations on the words and numbers received. The computer processes data by following a set of instructions stored in its memory. The set of instructions is called the program of instructions or simply the program. The program for doing a particular task, such as word processing, is also called the software or application software. When a particular task is completed, the computer is instructed to send the results to an output device, such as a printer or a monitor.

A note on terminology: We will use the term "computer" for personal computer, PC, microcomputer, desktop computer, and laptop computer. For the word processing example to be discussed, we will use a computer with keyboard, monitor, hard disk, and printer, known collectively as the hardware or the equipment used. Two types of software will be used, the disk operating system (DOS) for housekeeping and other operating instructions, and the application software for word processing.

Components

The case in which the computer is housed has a button or a switch to turn it on and off and outlets or ports for cables to connect it to the other components and to an electric outlet. It has one or more slots into which diskettes are inserted. The diskette, either 5–1/4 inches or 3–1/2 inches in diameter, serves as both input and output media for the computer. Input includes the DOS, the application software, and the data to be processed by the computer. The output consists of data that have been processed and are to be stored on diskette. Inside the case is a board containing the central processing unit (CPU) on a microchip and the random access memory (RAM). There are slots, called expansion slots, in which cards are inserted. The cards are hardware needed for the hard disk, the color monitor, and special programs such as those that make computers talk. Diskette drives that read and write data are the input and output devices in the back of the slots in which the diskettes are inserted. A hard disk with an associated disk drive, the input and output device that reads from and writes to the hard disk, is also inside the computer. Cables inside the case connect the different parts of the computer and a fan keeps the parts from overheating.

The keyboard is an input device, a device for sending information to the computer. The keyboard is similar to that on a typewriter; the keys for letters and numbers are in the same relative location as those on a typewriter. The computer keyboard has additional keys for performing special functions. An example of a special function key is the insert key. When this key is in the insert or edit mode, text can be inserted at the location of the cursor. There are also special keys that have different functions in different programs. These keys are called F or function keys and are used by themselves or in combination with other keys for such different commands as displaying a help screen with information about the program that we are running, underlining part of the text, or sending the text to the printer.

The monitor consists of a cathode ray tube on which text or pictures are displayed. The screen can be controlled for brightness and contrast, just like a television screen. The monitor is both an input and an output device. It is an input device when it accepts a message from a clicking device called a mouse or trackball. It is an output device when it displays information on the screen. Monitors come in varying screen sizes and in either monochrome or color. Color monitors vary in quality or resolution of image.

The printer is an output device that prints one line or a page at a time. Printers vary in both speed and quality of print produced. Other variables are the color of print produced and paper used. Printing can be on single sheets, continuous forms, envelopes, or labels with adhesive backing. Dot matrix printers are the least expensive. They are slower, noisier, and do not produce the high-quality print or illustrations of the more expensive laser printers.

Hard disk

A hard disk and its associated disk drive can store large amounts of information. Storage capacity is measured in megabytes or millions of characters. Hard disks with a capacity of a hundred or more megabytes are no longer unusual. Just like the diskette, the hard disk is an input device when data are read from it and an output device when data are written onto it. The hard disk, however, has a greater storage capacity and greater reading and writing speed than diskettes. Because of these advantages, the DOS, the application software packages, and the files produced on the computer are stored on hard disk rather than on diskettes. Backup copies are, or at least should be, stored on diskettes, as a safeguard against accidental erasure.

Screen character enlargement programs

These programs enable one to enlarge characters on the screen to one inch in height or even larger. J.C. DeWitt and others (see references at the end of this chapter) prepared a review of six such programs for IBM and IBM-compatible computers. While this review does not include the most recent programs, their criteria for evaluating screen character enlargement programs still apply. They are

- Ease of switching back and forth from word processing or other application programs to the character enlargement program;
- Ability to enlarge a line, column, or other portion of the screen;
- Choice of size, boldness, spacing, and color of characters and background.

The character enlargement programs are memory-resident; that is, they share RAM space with the DOS and the application program that we are running. We need to make sure that we have enough memory space for all three programs. We also need to make sure that the combination of keys used for invoking the screen character enlargement program does not conflict with a combination of keys used in the application program.

Speech synthesizers

Special hardware and software are needed to make our computer talk. A screen access program is the software that sends the signals displayed on the monitor to the speech synthesizer. The speech synthesizer can be in a box connected to the computer or on a card that fits into one of the computer's expansion slots. The screen access program is memory-resident. The screen access program that actuates the speech synthesizer is different from an application program. It works with the associated speech synthesizer to make the application program talk. When we wish to use a word processing program with a speech synthesizer, we call both the screen access program and the word processing program into memory. When these programs are ready to run, the computer will start talking. The computer reads aloud what is on the screen. This may be part of a document that we are keying in or a document stored on hard disk. Speech synthesizers range in quality of speech from very strange to sounding almost like a person. Synthetic speech can usually be varied in speed, volume, pitch, and other voice characteristics. The journal article by Meyers and Schreier (see references) evaluates commercially available screen access programs in terms of ease of installation and use and the following suggested desirable characteristics:

- Ability to move quickly to any part of the screen by specifying line number, portion of screen, or a specific word on the screen;
- Option of reading every word, number, and punctuation mark or spell out words or spell out the function of individual keys;
- Ability to read the menu and other lines above and below the space for keying in text or numbers;

- Use of a combination of keys that do not conflict with the same combination of keys used in application programs; and
- Enough memory left for the application program.

Braille input and output devices

For those of us who read and write braille, alternate computer input and output devices may be used. Instead of the typewriter-like keyboard, a seven-key braille keyboard on a braille input device may be used. Braille output devices either emboss braille characters on paper (hard-copy braille) or shape braille characters with the heads of pins (electronic, paperless, or refreshable braille). The person reading braille senses the configuration of dots in each braille cell, whether it is embossed or shaped by the heads of pins. Electronic braille output devices display one line of twenty to eighty braille cells at a time. When one line of braille cells has been read, another line can be displayed on command.

A point about the utility of screen character enlargement programs, speech synthesizers, and braille input and output devices: The use of programs with graphic user interface (GUI) is a new development in the computer field. While a GUI has advantages for sighted computer users, it presents a problem for users of screen enlargement programs and speech synthesizers. Most of these adaptive devices do not pick up GUI characters and therefore cannot be used for enlarging or reading them. Work is under way on adaptive devices that can handle a graphics user interface. IBM has announced the autumn 1992 availability of Screen Reader/2, a screen access program for speech synthesizers that also reads graphics characters.

Page scanners

A page scanner, also called an optical character reader, is an input device that translates print into signals that the computer can process. Page scanners vary in what they can scan and in the speed and accuracy of scanning. Some can scan only single sheets, while others can also scan pages from bound volumes. Some scanners have hand-held cameras or input units; others have cameras in a fixed location.

Page scanners and speech synthesizers can be purchased separately and attached to the computer or as a system with all of the components included. An example of the latter is the Kurzweil Personal Reader, made by Kurzweil Computer Products, a pioneer in reading machines for the blind (see resources).

Modems

We are not limited to working with data or programs that are stored on our diskettes or hard disk. We have potential access to files on other computers, including bulletin boards and commercial databases that will be discussed in this and the next chapter. To access data on other computers, we need to attach a modem to our computer and to a telephone line. The modem is a communication device that allows computer data to be sent over ordinary telephone lines. With the associated software it permits us to connect our computer with another computer. The modem will also dial the telephone number for us if we keep it in memory. Once we are linked to the other computer, we use it in the same way we use our own computer.

Computer operations

Let us go back to the central processing unit (CPU) and the random access memory (RAM). The RAM contains all the information that the computer needs for doing its job. This information consists of

- *The data.* The numbers or words and other characters translated as numbers that are to be processed. The initial data sent by the input device, data partially processed and shuttled back and forth between the CPU and the RAM, and data ready to be sent out of the computer via the output device are all stored in the RAM.
- *The application program.* The step-by-step instructions that tell the computer what to do with the data.
- *DOS.* The disk operating program that starts the computer and sends data and instructions back and forth between the RAM and the CPU, and to and from the RAM to the input and output devices.

The RAM is connected directly to the CPU, which is where the processing takes place, one step at a time. Complex operations on numbers or words translated as numbers are done as combinations of simple operations. The simple operations are additions, subtractions, multiplications, divisions, and comparisons of numbers. These operations are done at the rate of millions of operations per second.

When the computer is turned on, a copy of DOS is taken automatically from the hard disk and placed into RAM. DOS then checks for any computer malfunction. If none is found, it places a prompt on the screen indicating that everything is ready to go. Next, the application program to be used is selected from hard disk or diskette by keyboard command and the program is sent to RAM. When the program is set to run, data to be processed are sent to RAM from the keyboard or other input device. The processing of the data can now take place, since both the data and application program are in RAM. Under instruction from DOS, also in RAM, data and instructions to process the data are sent in and out of the CPU until the operation is complete and no additional instructions are sent from the input device. The processed data, the results of the operation, are sent to the output device selected by the user, again under the direction of DOS.

Computer applications

We will now describe several computer applications, along with the software application packages needed to perform these tasks. With the exception of word processing, we will not mention specific application programs. There are a number of software program reviews in magazines that give the pros and cons of the specific programs as well as their cost.

Word processing

Word processing is probably the first thing we will do with a computer. Let's begin by writing a letter on the computer, but this time let's do it right. We turn on the computer and get a C prompt, a C and a "greater than" sign. The C indicates that we are in the directory labelled C, which is the hard disk. The C prompt tells us the computer is ready to work for us. We request that a copy of the word processing program, WordPerfect

5.1, be sent to RAM so that we can use it for writing a letter. The command is C:\WP51. This tells the computer to go to a file called WP51. The 51 tells the computer that, in case we have more than one version of WordPerfect, we want version 5.1. We press the "Enter" key, which tells the computer to copy the file and send the copy to RAM. All messages must be keyed in and sent to the computer by depressing the "Enter" key, sometimes called the return key. We will now see the WordPerfect logo on the screen, followed by the editing screen. The editing screen is a blank screen, except for the cursor on the upper left of the screen and a line at the lower right that gives the document, page, line, and position of the cursor.

In the description that follows, some but by no means all of the features of this program are given. Before we prepare any document (the generic term for letters, reports, or anything else that we write), we have a number of formatting options. We can set the program for spacing, left, right, top, and bottom margins, line justification, and pagination. We can underline words, have them appear in bold characters, and change size and style of type font. The date of the document can be inserted automatically by depressing one of the function keys in combination with another key. After we have selected the formatting options, we key in or input the letter.

We can store and command the computer to insert unchanging parts of documents, such as our address and endings of letters. When we have completed keying in the letter, we use the spell checker to locate and correct errors in spelling. In this part of the process, the computer compares each word in the letter with words in its internally stored list of words. If it locates a word that is not in its list of words, it marks the word on the screen and usually suggests one or more words that we might have meant to type. We can select one of these words, select a word not on the list of suggested words, or decide to keep the word as originally typed. Words that we select will be automatically inserted into the text. Words not in the list of words can be added for use in subsequent spell checking. If the "mot juste" for expressing our thoughts escapes us, we can call on another part of the program, an internally stored thesaurus. We will find synonyms and near synonyms of words in the thesaurus, words that we can use in preference to the ones that we have used. At any point in keying in a document, we may decide to change things around a bit by moving a phrase, a sentence, or a paragraph. Function keys are used to send the completed document to the printer and print one or a designated number of copies. The document in electronic form can be saved or stored under a file name that we select. We can call for this document by file name and use part or all of it in other documents without having to key in the repeated information. The session with the word processing program is ended by exiting from the program. We can then either exit from the computer by signing off or call up another program.

Database management programs

Documents that we keep—correspondence, notes, magazine articles, bills—and information contained in these documents can be located with the aid of a database management program, which provides a guide to the location and the content of documents. These documents and this information may be physically stored inside the computer in electronic form or outside the computer on paper or diskette. The topic of locating items was introduced in chapter 1 when we dealt with locating items of clothing of a particular color; the topic will be dealt with further in chapter 3. Here we are primarily concerned with inputting information about individual documents into the computer and then searching for documents with specified information.

The documents in our example are magazine articles on leisure activities for visually disabled persons. We need to keep in mind that we have one file, the paper copies of the magazine articles. These articles are filed by accession number in file folders. The accession number is a unique number given to each document for identification and for filing. The following information for each document is input into the computer:

- Accession number;
- Bibliographic citation of document including author, title of article, title, volume, date, and pages of publication;
- Name of leisure activity;
- Need to modify leisure activity for visually impaired persons (yes or no);
- Physical effort entailed in activity (one of three defined levels);

- Mental effort entailed in activity (one of three defined levels); and
- Out-of-pocket cost of activity (one of three defined ranges).

Computer input of information about each document

The input, or record, for each magazine article is keyed in at the computer and under the direction of the database management program. This task is facilitated by having a blank form with all of the headings for the categories listed above. This form is called a template. The database management program is called up by its abbreviated name. A menu appears on the screen that lists choices of actions that can be performed when entering the program. The "add new items" or input choice is selected. A blank template will appear on the screen. Each appropriate category is filled in for that record, and, after it has been proofed for accuracy, the newly completed template is stored. In this way, the newly entered information about the document is incorporated into the file. This process is repeated for as many new documents as need to be input into the file. We then exit the file and the database management program.

Computer output or searching the file

The database management program is again called up. We select the "search" option from the initial menu. This generates a blank template on which we key in the terms needed in our search. We may, for example, search for a leisure activity with a high level (3) of mental effort, a low level (1) of physical effort, and a cost of less than fifty dollars. To conduct this search, we key in the appropriate numbers in the mental effort, physical effort, and cost categories. The computer then looks for leisure activities that have the specified characteristics. If such leisure activities are located, the corresponding completed templates are displayed on the screen, one at a time. Instead of displaying all of the information about each of the matching activities, only some of the information, for example, the name of the activity, may be displayed. Other output options are preparing paper copies of the search results on the printer or storing them on disk for subsequent processing. The search is terminated by exiting the program and then exiting the computer, unless another program is to be run.

Searching remote databases

Technology now permits us to sit at our computer and use the programs and files stored on another computer. The other computer may be located next door, across the country, or in another country. Unless we are addressing another computer in a local network in which two or more computers are linked on a more or less permanent basis, we will need a modem and a voice-grade telephone line to connect our computer to the other computer. Why would we want to use information on somebody else's computer? To answer this question, we will look at two commercial services, Prodigy and BRS, that offer information for a fee. Both of these commercial services allow us to use their computer from our computer when the two computers are connected with modems and a telephone line.

Prodigy. Prodigy provides a wide variety of information for a flat fee of about thirteen dollars a month. There are no long-distance phone charges if Prodigy has a telephone number in our community. A simple protocol and our password connects us to Prodigy. The initial screen gives news headlines backed by fuller stories displayed upon request. Keying in words from a list of key words will get us to different parts of the system. Here are some of the things that we can find with Prodigy:

- National and international news
- Stock market quotations
- Articles from a general encyclopedia
- Consumer product reviews
- Lists of hotels, restaurants, and other travel information
- Film reviews
- Restaurant reviews
- Electronic messages sent to and received from other subscribers of Prodigy

- Information exchange about computers and other topics via electronic bulletin boards
- Games to play at the computer

Prodigy also lists and briefly describes items from catalogs of merchandise from a variety of merchants. Items can be ordered at the computer and paid for with a credit card. For those of us who find shopping in stores either difficult or less than fun, shopping at the computer is an alternative.

Signing off the system is accomplished with a couple of simple keystrokes. A computer has to have a specified amount of memory and a color monitor with graphic card to use Prodigy as intended. Prodigy has a graphics user interface that refers its user to a screen access program that is intended to work with speech synthesizers.

BRS. BRS is an example of a commercial information service but, unlike Prodigy, it is intended for a special rather than a general audience. It is used primarily by students, researchers, doctors, teachers, and other professionals to identify publications on topics of interest. BRS has databases in medicine, agriculture, sociology, chemistry, and many other fields. These databases provide access to the contents of magazine articles, patents, reports, conference proceedings, and other research publications. The databases may be searched by author name, organization name, subject, date, language, type of publication, and other types of access points. The cost of searching BRS databases varies with the specific database searched, the amount of time spent in searching the database, the number of references selected, and the time of day of the search. We can easily spend twenty or more dollars for a search. BRS searchers using their own computers need to subscribe to the service. Payment of the subscription fee will get us a password to enter the system and instruction manuals for using it.

Before we can search BRS we need to connect our computer to the BRS computer. A telecommunication network such as Sprintnet is typically used to save on long-distance telephone charges. The BRS system is requested and, when connected, is unlocked with our passwords. Then we request a database to be searched and key in the search statement. The search statement consists of author, subject, and other access points. The computer is asked to identify documents with a specified combination of search terms.

The computer's initial response is the number of documents that meet the search specification. If the number is too small or too large, we can modify the search statement. When the number of identified publications appears satisfactory, we request identifying information about these documents. All or any part of the information in the database about a document can be obtained. The information consists of the bibliographic citation, with or without a summary or abstract of the publication. Some databases even include the full text of each publication. Information about identified documents can be sent to our printer or to our hard disk. The identified documents can be sorted by author, date, or other arrangement before being sent to us. We can continue with another search of the same database, request another database and search it, or sign off the system with a simple protocol.

The book by Glossbrenner (see references), available from NLS in recorded form, includes a more detailed description of a number of remote databases.

Other application programs

We might want to consider desktop publishing for producing newsletters or other publications that need to look good. Desktop publishing programs allow us to vary type size and fonts for headlines or for highlighting text, to arrange text in columns, and to insert illustrations. Some of these tasks can be done with word processing programs but not as well as with desktop publishing programs specifically intended for this purpose.

If the newsletter goes to a large number of people and if the names on our mailing list change often, we might consider a mailing list program. Again, the word processing program can be used for typing and sorting, but large and frequently changing mailing lists might make a specialized mailing list program desirable.

Businesses need to keep complex financial records of income and expenses for tax and other purposes. Accounting programs are available to keep such records for businesses and for individuals as well. Some of these programs permit electronic transfer of funds and thus save one from having to write and mail checks.

Obtaining computer hardware and software

Before we think seriously about obtaining a computer with the needed adaptive devices and software, we should have a good idea of what we want to do with it. This is not only necessary to convince ourselves, our employer, or the state agency for the blind to spend the money but also to select the computer, adaptive devices, and software that are best for us.

The cost of equipment has gone down over the past few years but is still high. Here are some suggestions for the buyer.

If at all possible, try out the equipment and software before buying. Someone in town may let us try out his or her equipment; computer bulletin boards or local dealers might be able to connect us with such a person. Some computer manufacturers offer a discount to disabled persons. Low-interest loans may be available to us. A lease-purchase plan is another possibility; under such a plan we own the equipment upon payment of a predetermined number of monthly payments.

While mail-order firms may give us the best prices, they do not necessarily give us the best deals. A local merchant might charge a bit more, but the extra cost may be worth it if he installs the equipment in our home and responds to questions that we will be sure to have. Also, payment by credit card is recommended to give us recourse for nonreceived or nonworking items.

Two recommended readings on the topic are the Hadley School for the Blind's *Introduction to Microcomputers*, a text on cassette for their course on microcomputers, and *The Second Beginner's Guide to Personal Computers for the Blind and Visually Impaired* published by the National Braille Press (see references).

References

DeWitt, J.C., E.M. Schreier, and J.D. Leventhal. "A Guide to Selecting Large Print/Enhanced Image Computer Access Hardware/Software for Persons with Low Vision." *Journal of Visual Impairment and Blindness* 82(1988):432-442.

Glossbrenner, Alfred. *The Complete Handbook of PC Communication*; 3rd ed. New York: St. Martin's Press, 1990. (RC 31483)

Introduction to Microcomputers, rev. ed. Winnetka, IL: Hadley School for the Blind, 1990.
      For information about correspondence courses on microcomputers, call the school at 1-800-323-4238 or write to 700 Elm Street, Winnetka, IL 60093.

Meyers, A., and E. Schreier. "An Evaluation of Speech Access Programs." *Journal of Visual Impairment and Blindness* 84(1990): 26-38.

The Second Beginner's Guide to Personal Computers for the Blind and Visually Impaired, 2nd ed. Boston: National Braille Press, 1987.
      Available in print, braille, or on cassette from the publisher at 88 St. Stephen Street, Boston, MA 02115.

Resources

BRS
Maxwell Online, Inc.
8000 Westpark Drive
McLean, VA 22102
1-800-289-4277

Kurzweil Computer Products
185 Albany Street
Cambridge, MA 02139
1-800-343-0311

Prodigy
Prodigy Services Company
P.O. Box 791
White Plains, NY 10601
1-800-284-5933

3. Personal information management systems

When we wake up in the morning, the alarm clock tells us it is time to get up. The radio announcer informs us of the weather for the day and we dress accordingly. The teacher or boss tells us what is expected of us and we react to this information. All of us are constantly receiving and reacting to information. We do this with the aid of what can be called our personal information management system or PIM for short. PIM receives, acts upon, and stores information. Every day we are subjected to, some say bombarded with, messages from many different sources—radio, television, newspapers, magazines, bosses, teachers, family members, and friends. It is difficult for us to pay attention to all of these messages, let alone make use of them. A point of terminology: We are using the words "information" and "message" interchangeably for whatever persons may tell us in person, over the phone, in writing addressed specifically to us, or in writing addressed to many persons.

We need a mechanism for screening us from unwanted information. PIM performs this function, but not flawlessly. There are times when our PIM either does not screen us from unwanted information or screens us from wanted information. PIM also plays a role in gathering, organizing, storing, and retrieving information. We gather information first by selecting the source and then by querying the source. The information may be put to immediate use, typically for making a decision. We may decide to keep the information for possible later use. Keeping the information means organizing and storing it. The information may be on paper, cassette, computer disk, or in our head. Organization may be formal, such as papers neatly arranged in file folders and filed by topic, or it may also be informal—papers piled at random on the dining room table.

In this chapter I will discuss ways of gathering information from persons and from publications, alternate ways of reading, and ways of organizing information.

Gathering information

There are two basic ways of gathering information. We may ask someone who is likely to know, or we may look for the information in a book or other publication.

When we need to gather or collect information—that is, when we have a question—the most convenient way to get an answer is to ask someone. It is more convenient than looking for the answer in a publication because it permits us to interact with the person: we can reword our question if we think that it was misunderstood; we can ask the person to reword the answer if we do not understand it. Such interaction is not possible when we look in publications for answers to questions.

If we know a person who is knowledgeable on the subject, we merely contact that person and ask him or her our question. If we do not know such a person, we have to take the preliminary step of identifying such a person. Two ways of doing this are to attend a meeting of an organization or to consult an electronic bulletin board.

Attending conferences or meetings of organizations

Conferences or meetings of organizations are planned events at which people with common interests get together for a variety of reasons, two of which are to exchange information and to have fun. We might attend a conference of an organization of the blind to find persons who are knowledgeable about the job market, adaptive equipment for using computers, or any other topics of interest to people with visual disabilities. Most of us enjoy going to a conference. It gives us a chance to get away from our everyday routine. We see old friends and meet new ones, go to parties, and, last but not least, give and obtain information.

When attending a conference, we exchange information at formal sessions where papers are presented; at exhibits, where we can see new products and talk to vendors about them; at parties; in bars; in the corridors of the conference hotel; or wherever else conference participants get together. A conference is a good setting for information exchange because it provides a forum for people interested and knowledgeable in a particular subject field.

Using electronic bulletin boards

Another way of locating knowledgeable persons in a given field who are willing to share their knowledge is to consult an electronic bulletin board. The bulletin board is operated by either a local or national group, people who share a common interest. This interest is not limited to computers but can be, for example, gardening, literature, or protecting the environment. We can consult the public library for information about local and national electronic bulletin boards. We need a password and knowledge of the sign-on routine to connect our computer to the computer with the electronic bulletin board. Bulletin board questions or messages may be addressed to anyone who consults the bulletin board or to one or more specific individuals. Electronic bulletin boards provide a mechanism for identifying persons knowledgeable in a subject field as well as for obtaining answers to specific questions.

Getting information from publications

There are times when we cannot or do not wish to locate a person willing and able to answer our question. We may not want to reveal our ignorance about a subject or reveal an interest in a subject for proprietary or other reasons. When that happens, we look for the answer in a publication, such as a book, a magazine article, or a newspaper article. These publications are kept in libraries and perhaps in our personal collection along with notes, bills, and correspondence.

Libraries are institutions charged with gathering, organizing, storing, and retrieving publications and information contained in publications. These are also some of the functions of our PIM. The difference is one of size and complexity necessitated by the much larger size of a library than a personal collection. We will now look at how we can locate publications in a library. PIMs will be dealt with later in the chapter.

Identifying and locating a book in a library

For our example, we will visit the local public library. The steps in identifying and locating a book will be the same in school, college, university, and other types of libraries. The public library, unlike other libraries, is charged with serving all the residents of a specified geographic area, including residents who are visually disabled.

Our first task in the library will be to check whether a specific book is in the library collection and, if it is, to locate it and borrow it for home use. We need to follow these steps to complete this task:

1. Find out if the book is in the library's collection by looking it up in the library catalog.
2. If the book is in the collection, find out where it is located in the library.
3. Pick up the book from the shelves.
4. Charge out the book for home use.

Help in performing these tasks may be obtained from the library staff. For steps 1 and 2, finding out whether the book is in the library collection and determining its location in the library, we consult the library catalog. The library catalog, in card trays and/or on computer, is the guide to the location of publications in the library. Each publication that the library acquires—each book, magazine, videotape, audiotape, or other separate publication—is listed in the library catalog.

We will begin by looking at a catalog in card form. The basic unit of the card catalog is the individual catalog card. For a book, the card lists the author or authors, title, publisher, year of publication, and, if applicable, the edition. Also on each card is a code that tells us where in the library the book is located, if it is in its appointed spot on the shelf. The individual cards are filed alphabetically. Cards for each book are filed under the name of its author or authors, its title, and its subject or subjects. The word or phrase under which we need to look to locate a catalog card for a given book is called either the filing point or the access point.

Consider looking at a catalog card for a book as looking at a surrogate or substitute for the book. The catalog card contains information that will help us decide whether or not we want to look at the book itself.

36

The location information tells us where to look for the book. The location code, the "call number," consists of a unique combination of letters and numbers for each copy of a book in a library. The call number places books on the same subject with each other and books on related subjects near each other. The call number also differentiates multiple copies of the same book so that we will not be charged for a book not returned by another borrower. In the card catalog, the cards for each book—author, title, and subject cards—are arranged in a single, alphabetical file or in two alphabetical files, the author file and the title and subject file.

More and more library catalogs are now in electronic form for searching by computer terminals located in the library. Some libraries have converted their entire card catalog to electronic form; others have kept the card form for older publications, which means users must search both card and electronic catalogs to identify all publications on a subject or by an author in the library collection. The information provided for each book or other publication is usually the same in both forms of catalogs.

We search the card catalog by removing from its cabinet the card tray that includes the cards with the needed filing point and scanning the alphabetically arranged cards by author, title, or subject. We note the call number of the wanted item and are ready for the next step, the retrieval of the item.

We search the library catalog on computer by keying in the selected filing point at the computer terminal. The computer then tells us how many, if any, publications in the library are listed under that filing point. We request a display of identifying information about the selected items, including their call numbers. This information can be printed out for us if there is a printer at the computer terminal.

Now for our first search of the catalog. We are looking for a recent book by Nathan Miller about American spies. Our clues for this search are the name of the author, a subject, and an indication of the date of publication. We do not know the title of the book. A search under Miller, Nathan, identifies a 1989 publication by Nathan Miller entitled *Spying for America*. We think that is the book we want. We looked for this book by the name of the author because the author is the best filing point or access point to use if we are reasonably sure of having the right name. A search by title is next best if we are reasonably sure that we have an exact title and if the title is not too general, such as *English Literature*.

The phrase "English literature" would, most likely, yield not only the book that we want to identify but many other books as well.

If we are not sure of the author's name or the title of the book, or if the search is for any books on a topic, we would use the subject as the access point. This is usually a more difficult search because a subject may be called by different names. We need to know what word or phrase is used in the catalog to describe this subject to find books on the subject. In our example, a spy may be called a secret agent, a spook, a CIA agent, or a KGB agent. We may want to look for books on this subject under any of these terms. The library cannot file books on this subject under all possible words we can think of, so how do we find the word or phrase that is used in the catalog to designate a particular topic? Rephrasing this question in words that librarians would use, under what subject headings should we search? To help us conduct subject searches, librarians have provided directions that give us a map of the territory. These directions are called "see" references and "see also" references. For example, "Spying—See Espionage" tells us to look under "Espionage" for publications about spying. "Espionage—See also Intelligence service" tells us that additional publications on topics related to espionage will be found under the subject heading "Intelligence service."

Back to our search for Nathan Miller's book. We memorize, copy, or print out the book's call number, depending on confidence in our memory and on whether a computer printer is available. Next, we pick out the book from the shelves by looking for it under its call number. If the book is on the shelves, we take it to the circulation desk and charge it out for home use. If the book is not on the shelves, we can ask at the circulation desk for its whereabouts. It may be charged out or it may be at the bindery getting a new cover. We can request to be notified upon the book's return and have it set aside for our use. The book may be lost or stolen. Another copy of the book may then be purchased, unless it is no longer for sale. Most book titles go out of print within a few years of their publication and can no longer be purchased from book stores or publishers. Such books may be borrowed from another library under a procedure called interlibrary loan. Borrowing a book on interlibrary loan takes one or more weeks and may entail a charge of several dollars.

Locating magazine articles on a subject

Suppose that we are interested in information on a topic that is too new to be described in a book. The topic that we want to investigate is the artificial eye. What we want is not information on spy satellites but on a device that, if and when perfected, will enable a blind person to see. A friend of ours mentioned that research is being done on this topic and we want to learn more about it. We look for articles on the topic in magazines. Magazine articles on a topic are identified with the aid of magazine indexes. Just as the library catalog is the tool for locating books and other separate publications in the library, magazine indexes are tools for finding articles in issues of magazines. Searches of magazine indexes by author or by subject yield magazine articles that are identified by their bibliographic citations, which consist of the author and title of the article; the title of the magazine; and the volume, date, and pages where the article appears. Computer-searched indexes, also called databases, to medical, technical, and other specialized magazines were mentioned in chapter 2 in the section on BRS, a commercial information service. Here we are interested in an index that covers general magazines, the type that we can buy at a newsstand.

As with library catalogs, magazine indexes come in both printed and electronic forms. The one that we select for our search is the General Magazine Index, a computer-searched index that includes publications such as *Newsweek*, *The Atlantic*, and the *New York Times*. Several years of the index are on a compact disk—called a CD-ROM (compact disk read only memory). The instructions for searching the index are posted at the computer terminal. We use the given combination of keystrokes to select the General Magazine Index, to locate the appropriate access point "Eye, artificial," and to print out identifying information about the seven potentially relevant articles that are retrieved. For some magazine articles, although not for those we retrieve, the entire text is stored in the computer and can be printed at the terminal.

Two other differences exist between commercial databases, such as BRS, and indexes on CD-ROM. First, the CD-ROM is in the library, while commercial databases are in remote locations and on someone else's computer. Second, the CD-ROM search is free, while the remote database search typically entails a charge to the user that may be twenty dollars or more for a search.

The seven articles identified in the search are in three different magazines and one newspaper, the *New York Times*. We check the library catalog for the location of identified titles, just as we did in the book search. We find six of the articles on the shelves and read them. The seventh article is in a magazine not in the library; we order a photocopy on interlibrary loan. The procedure is similar to borrowing a book on interlibrary loan; it takes a week or more, at a typical cost to the user of several dollars.

Other reasons for using public libraries

Most public libraries have books of fiction and nonfiction in regular print, large print, and on cassette. The books on cassette may be sample collections of books from the National Library Service for the Blind and Physically Handicapped (NLS) or commercial publications. In addition to providing reading material, the public library may provide the following services to visually disabled persons:

- A reading area where a sighted companion can read aloud to us without disturbing others;
- Retrieval of publications from the shelves;
- Photocopies of publications;
- A list of volunteer readers and braillers;
- Reading short passages of text;
- Answering questions, either in person or over the telephone.

Public libraries also offer a variety of programs directly or indirectly related to reading. Book discussion groups, lectures, and workshops are examples of programs in which visually disabled persons can participate.

Reading

We have located magazine articles and need to read them to satisfy the information need that brought us to the library. How do we read these articles or other reading matter when we have a specific purpose in mind? The "how to read" in this question has two meanings that concern us. It may refer to what portion or portions of the publication we read and how thoroughly we do so, or it may refer to how we sense the words that we read, whether by sight, by hearing, or by touch. We will call the former the reading strategy and the latter the reading method.

Reading strategy

Chances are that if we read every word of every publication that we need to read, we would never get the job done. There is actually no need to read every word if we have figured out ahead of time why we need to read it. The plan for reading a publication is called the reading strategy.

We will consider reading strategy in terms of reading a magazine article. The typical magazine article includes the following components:

- A summary or abstract that tells briefly what the article is about;
- An introduction that sets the stage of the article and summarizes previous thinking or work on this subject;
- The body of the article—the presentation of the findings or the argument—perhaps with possible applications;
- Conclusions to highlight the contribution of the article;
- Charts, tables, photographs, and other illustrations for matter best presented in graphic form; and
- References to the publications used and cited in the article.

The first step in the reading strategy is to determine the purpose of the reading—the "why." There are many reasons for reading an article, but we will consider the two most likely—a desire for background information on a subject and a desire for specific facts. For both reasons, we need to find out whether or not a particular magazine article is likely to have the needed information. We can usually determine this by reading the abstract or summary.

For background information we typically read the introduction, the conclusion, the headings of the sections of the article, the headings of illustrations, and parts or all of the body of the article.

For locating a fact or facts in the article, we read the headings of sections and illustrations to determine where the facts are likely to be reported and then read that portion. Again, not every word or even every section of the publication needs to be read.

Reading method

The second aspect of how one reads deals with the way we sense the symbols that we read. We read print with our eyes, we hear print that is read to us, or we read raised characters with our fingertips. Not all of us are capable of using these three basic methods of reading. Our eyesight may not permit us to read print, even in enlarged form. We may not have learned braille. But to provide an overview of reading methods, the three basic methods will be compared in terms of three factors that have a bearing on the selection of the reading method, if we are given a choice. These factors are

1. The need to move from one part to other parts of a publication. Looking for a telephone number of a person entails looking in only one place, the alphabetic listing by last name. Reading a magazine article, on the other hand, may entail looking in different portions of the article. We call the ability to go to different portions of a publication with a particular reading method its *ease of navigation*.
2. The amount of time that we can spend reading without discomfort we call the *reading comfort* of the method. While we may be able to look up a telephone number with a relatively uncomfortable reading method, say using a hand-held magnifier, we would not want to use this method for lengthy reading.
3. Photographs and other illustrations are an important part of some publications, and reading methods differ in their ability to display illustrations. This ability is called the *reading illustrations* factor of the reading method.

Reading publications in large print

Large print characters are 14 points or greater in height. (A point is 1/72 of an inch, so a publication in 18-point type is printed with characters 1/4 inch high.) Many fiction and nonfiction books are now published in both regular and large print. The *Reader's Digest* is an example of a magazine that is also published in large print. The *New York Times Large Print Weekly* is a portion of the newspaper published in large print. Dictionaries, encyclopedias, thesauri, and other reference books are published in large print. Most public libraries have fiction, nonfiction, and reference books in this form. A reference book called *Large Type Books in Print* lists commercially published books in large print. This reference book may be found in libraries or bookstores.

Large-print books, for those of us who are able to read them, rate high on all three reading method factors: ease of navigation, reading comfort, and reading illustrations.

Enlarging print with nonelectronic magnifying devices

For some of us, large print is not big enough to read or the publications that we need are not available in large print. We may be able to use devices for enlarging print to the size that we can read. As persons with limited vision, we differ not only in how much or how little we can see, but also in the type of magnifying devices available to us that make the most of our sight. There are many magnifying devices to choose from. Magnifying glasses can be hand-held, mounted in eyeglass frames, attached to eyeglasses, or mounted on a stand. These glasses magnify print by a factor of two (2X) or higher. A magnifying factor of 6 or even higher is available for some magnifying glasses. We must keep in mind that the greater the magnification, the smaller the area that is being magnified. A sixfold illuminated magnifying device mounted in what looks like a flashlight may make characters big enough for us to read but will only permit us to see a few characters at a time. Magnifying glasses on a stand, in eyeglass frames, or mounted on eyeglasses leave our hands free, an advantage when we need to read and write at the same time.

All of these devices are relatively inexpensive, costing from less than $10 to about $150. Magnifying glasses can be purchased from a local drugstore, a hobby store, a mail-order house specializing in equipment for the visually disabled, a low-vision optometrist, or a low vision clinic. We may find it worthwhile to visit a low vision optometrist or a low-vision clinic, where we can try and compare a variety of devices until we find the one that is best for us.

Magnifying devices are used primarily for reading restaurant menus, telephone numbers, outlines of lecture notes, or other short items. Nonelectronic magnifying devices rate low on ease of navigation and reading comfort. They rate high on reading illustrations because we can use them for reading or viewing photographs and anything else that can be enlarged.

Closed circuit television (CCTV) reading machines

CCTV reading machines are the top of the line of magnifying devices. They come in either desktop or portable models. The desktop model consists of a movable platform, a television camera, a television monitor, and an illuminating device. The reading material, either a single sheet or a page in a book, is placed on the movable platform. The platform, which is illuminated, can be moved up or down or left to right to place the different portions of the page that are to be read under the television camera. The image taken by the television camera is projected onto the television monitor.

Instead of a television camera mounted on a stand, the portable CCTV reading machine has a hand-held television camera that is placed over the reading matter. The image then appears on a monitor, as with the desktop model. For portable CCTV reading machines a small hand-held monitor may be used. The monitor of a television set also may be used if its resolution is sufficiently high. It is best to try this out first, since blurry characters on a hazy background do not make for good reading. Degree of magnification is controlled by a single knob, as are focusing, brightness, and contrast. The polarity of the image (black on white or white on black) can be changed with a switch. CCTV reading machines may have the following options:

- Size of monitor
- Magnification up to sixty times

- Monochrome or color monitor
- Black, green, or amber monochrome screen

The cost of this equipment ranges from about $1,500 to $3,500.

The CCTV reading machine that I have used daily for the past four years has not needed any repair or maintenance. Even the light bulb that came with the machine has not burned out. I find that I can read with my CCTV for about two hours at one time. After that, my eyes get tired and I may see things that are not there and not see things that are there. A cautionary note: I have learned to move the platform on which the reading material rests slowly and smoothly to avoid the symptoms of seasickness brought on by fast and jerky motion.

Anything that can be placed under the machine's television camera can be projected on the screen and can, therefore, be read. However, very large or very thick books, such as some atlases, do not fit under the television camera of the desktop model, and books that have narrow inner margins and that cannot lie flat on the reading platform may present reading problems because the characters near the inner margin are likely to be distorted.

The material read can be highlighted or otherwise marked, because one can write as well as read with this machine. Pencil markings can be seen on the screen unless they are too near bold print or other brightly illuminated areas. Portable models can be used in the classroom and at meetings, or even taken to stores for identifying labels. CCTV reading machines rate high on ease of navigation and reading illustrations and medium for reading comfort.

Enlarging characters on a computer monitor

Chances are that if we use a computer the characters on the monitor are too small for us to read. We can resolve this problem in several ways. We can use a monitor with a screen of twenty-five or more inches, we can attach a magnifying device to our screen, we can wear magnifying eyeglasses, or we can install a software program that enlarges characters on the screen. A twenty-five-inch monitor or a magnifying device placed in front of a thirteen-inch monitor will nearly double the size of each character on the screen. The advantage of the larger monitor, the magnifying device, and the eyeglasses is that the screen will still display twenty-five lines with eighty characters per line, which is the number of characters on a standard computer screen. Most application programs—the word processing, database management, and other software programs that we are likely to use—assume that we have space for this number of lines and characters on our screen. If either one or the combination of these options works for us, that is probably the way to go.

The next option to consider is a character enlargement program. These programs were discussed in chapter 2 and can be used as a supplement as well as a substitute for the other options mentioned. How do large characters on a computer monitor measure on our three aspects of reading? Ease of navigation depends in part on the program used but is generally rated as medium. Reading comfort is also medium. The reading illustrations factor is low because most of the screen character enlargement programs available in 1992 do not project graphics on the monitor.

Printing notes in large characters

We may need to consult readable notes when we are away from our computer or reading machines, such as a list of items to buy at the supermarket or the outline of an oral presentation we have to give at work, in school, or at a club. The tedious way of writing readable notes is to take a felt-tipped pen or other writing tool that makes thick marks and draw one character after another. A better way is now available: One can type notes on the computer and print them out in characters of one inch or more in height. Commercial programs that cost about $50 will do this.

We key in our notes on the keyboard, one character at a time, until we have completed a letter-size page. Then we print the page on a dot matrix printer in about two minutes. The next page cannot be keyed in until the first page is printed. Using a laser printer with large type fonts is even faster and more efficient. We key in the notes just as we would key in a letter or any other document. Then we format what we have keyed into large print and instruct the printer to print one or more copies. A laser printer offers faster input, better quality print, ability to format documents already in the computer into large print, and faster output. We do not have to wait to type a second page while the first page is printed on the laser printer. We can prepare all of the pages of a document, then print them all. Also, we can take any document on the computer and re-format it to large print without having to key it in a second time.

Reading by listening to tape recordings

Tape recorders are used by visually disabled persons for writing and reading. We record notes and later listen to them. We also listen to tapes recorded by others, be they our readers or professional narrators.

Here are some features of tape recorders that we should consider if we do a lot of recording and if we listen to NLS books on cassettes. The tape recorders should

- Play and record at half of commercial speed as well as at commercial tape recording speed;
- Play and record on two tracks per cassette side;
- Permit tone indexing (the insertion of a beep to mark a passage of text, described later in this chapter);
- Record at fast forward for use in voice indexing (also discussed later in this chapter);
- Play at variable speeds, either faster or slower than the original recording;
- Have tactile marking on control keys; and
- Operate on house current or on batteries that are rechargeable by plugging the tape recorder into an electric outlet.

The APH 3-5104 tape recorder, the Handi-Cassette recorder, can be purchased from the American Printing House for the Blind for about $130. The recorder has all of the features listed above. The charge on the rechargeable battery lasts for about eight hours and is recharged by plugging the tape recorder into an electric outlet for about eight hours. The variable speed control makes it possible to listen to recordings at either slower or faster than normal speed. A pitch adjustment device is used to compensate for the higher or lower pitch at a faster or slower speed.

NLS lends users of its service tape players (but not tape recorders) for playing NLS books on cassette. Other tape players and tape recorders with some of the features listed are available from mail-order houses that specialize in products for visually disabled persons.

NLS is the major source of recreational reading in recorded form, as we will discuss in chapter 5. But one person's leisure reading may be another person's school reading. Students will find in the NLS collection classics of history, English and American literature, and many current books on a wide variety of topics useful in high school or college courses.

Another source for recorded books and books in electronic form is Recording for the Blind (RFB). RFB is a private philanthropic organization with a collection of about 79,000 recorded books on all subjects. Recorded books from RFB are free except for a one-time $25 fee.

As registered users we call to order a recorded book. If the book we request is in the RFB tape collection, a copy on cassettes will be sent to us promptly. If the book is not in the collection, RFB will record it for us, but it will take one or more months to get the cassette copy. To get a title recorded, we send RFB two print copies of the book, one for the narrator, the other for the person who monitors the recording to check the accuracy of the reading. The printed copies of the book will be returned to us with the cassettes. We may keep the book on cassette for a year or longer.

A new service of RFB is the sale of books on computer diskettes. Textbooks and reference books, such as a dictionary, can be bought in this form. These books can be read aloud with the aid of a speech synthesizer, a computer output device that was described in chapter 2.

Associated Services for the Blind is another philanthropic organization that, among other things, records magazines for blind persons. The recording may be of a single magazine or several magazines on one topic. An example of the latter is the recording of two personal computer magazines on cassette. A small fee is charged to recover part of the cost of the service. The recorded version of the monthly personal computer magazines is distributed about three months after the appearance of the printed magazines.

NLS also distributes recorded magazines but uses flexible disks rather than cassettes as the recording medium. NLS users can subscribe free of charge to magazines such as *The Atlantic*, *Harper's*, or *American Heritage*. Special record players are needed to read these magazines, which play at about eight revolutions per minute. NLS makes long-term loans of record players that play at that speed.

We may need to have a publication recorded, perhaps because the wait for RFB service is too long or because it is a magazine article, which falls outside the service provided by RFB. When we use our own readers, it is a good idea to give them written instructions or guidelines to help them record text in the way that we find most useful. Suggested guidelines for readers follow in table 1.

Reading by listening to tape recordings rates high for reading comfort. We can listen to recorded reading for hours on end and can take notes by recording them on a second tape recorder. A tape is intended to be read from beginning to end and therefore rates low for ease of navigation, although voice-indexed tape recordings rate medium for ease of navigation. A low rating is given for ease of viewing illustrations because illustrations must be described by the narrator.

Reading by listening to talking computers

Another reading option is listening to a computer talk. This option makes it possible not only to read text now in our computer but, as with the screen character reading programs, also any publication that has been captured in electronic form. As we noted in chapter 2, page scanners can be used to convert print into electronic signals, which in turn can be read with speech synthesizers. Speech synthesizers also read aloud computer input from the keyboard and thus provide immediate feedback for error correction.

Ease of navigation is considered medium for this method of reading. The method is rated high in reading comfort because, like listening to tape recordings, no eye strain occurs. It is rated low for reading illustrations because most programs available in 1992 cannot read graphics.

Reading braille

Reading braille consists of sensing combinations of raised dots with one's fingertips. The basic unit of braille is a combination of dots formed in a six-dot cell. Each unique combination of dots stands for a letter of the alphabet, a number, or a punctuation mark, and, depending on the grade

Table 1. Suggested guidelines for readers

1. Begin the recording with the complete bibliographic citation of the passage of text that will be read. For a book, this is the author, title, publisher, edition if applicable, date, and pages recorded. For a magazine article, it is the author, title of article, title of magazine, volume, year, and pages recorded.

2. Read the page number at the beginning of each new page.

3. Spell out names of authors.

4. Give headings of tables, graphs, and other illustrations but do not describe the contents.

5. Give number of items in the bibliography but do not read the individual citations.

6. It is all right to cough or to mispronounce a word. A perfect rendition of the text is not required or expected. The one and only function of the reading is to convey information.

7. However, reading should not sound as though the reader is about to fall asleep, as this will have a sleep-inducing effect on the listener.

8. Say "end of text" when this is the case.

9. Rewind the cassette at the end of the reading.

10. Start a new magazine article or a new section from a book on a new cassette.

11. Label the cassette in large letters with the name of the author and the date of the publication.

of braille used, words and parts of words. Three ways in which braille may differ will be mentioned since they have an effect on the three factors used for evaluating reading methods. The first variable is the number of abbreviations used. Grade 1 uses no abbreviations. Every character is assigned a unique combination of dots. In Grade 2 and Grade 3 braille, combinations of dots are used to designate characters as well as frequently used words and parts of words. Grade 3 has the most codes for abbreviations. All things being equal, the greater the number of abbreviations in the grade of braille, the fewer the number of braille characters that we need to write or read and, therefore, the faster the writing and reading. Braille also comes in two sizes, standard and jumbo. The larger characters of jumbo braille, intended for people whose fingertips are insufficiently sensitive to sense characters in standard braille, are probably slower to read.

The third braille variable is the physical format of the braille. It can either be embossed on paper, that is to say on hard copy, or it can be stored in electronic form on disk or cassette, to be displayed only when it is to be read. The latter form is called electronic, paperless, or refreshable braille. We mentioned this form in the discussion of computer input and output devices. Some electronic braillers can be used as either stand-alone devices or as computer input and output devices. The input device of an electronic brailler includes a seven-key braille keyboard. Its output device produces either synthesized speech or paperless braille or both. Paperless braille displays one line of twenty to eighty braille cells at a time. The braille dots in each braille cell are formed by raised heads of pins. The braille reader senses these raised heads of pins with his fingers. When the reading of one line of braille is completed, another line can be displayed.

The advantages of braille over other reading methods are summarized in an article by Lauer (see references). They include the ability to take, read, and file notes and to obtain exact spellings of names and other words that are sometimes unclear in recordings. It is possible to braille charts, maps, and other illustrations as embossed dots. Paper braille can be scanned more easily than recordings. However, it should be noted that braille is usually both difficult and time-consuming to learn, when one learns it past childhood. The speed of reading braille depends on what one reads, the grade of braille read, and the size of the braille characters read.

Paper braille rates high on ease of navigation because one can browse paper braille and scan it for passages of text the same way we do printed books. Braille in electronic form is rated as medium on ease of navigation because it is more difficult to get around in a publication in this format. Reading comfort is considered high for paper braille and medium for braille in electronic form. Braille on paper, like a book, can be read anywhere. This is also true of electronic braille but the limited number of characters displayed at one time suggests a medium rating on this factor. Ease of using illustrations is rated as medium for paper braille because illustrations are limited to what can be embossed. It is rated low for electronic braille because of an additional limitation: since only one line is displayed at a time, illustrations have to be limited to one line.

Conclusions on reading methods

As suggested in the article by Lauer, no single reading method is best for all the different types of reading one does. The choice of reading method is also circumscribed by whether or not one has any useful sight and by one's proficiency with braille. A summary of reading methods in terms of the three reading factors is presented in table 2. All things being equal, reading by listening to either human or synthetic speech is most suitable for lengthy readings without illustrations. If we have some usable sight, the CCTV reading machine is the best reading method for locating needed portions of text and for reading illustrations.

Other aspects of seeking and recording information

It may no longer be possible for us to read a printed daily newspaper, but we can read part of the paper in a different form. Prodigy, the computer-based commercial information service described in chapter 2, displays on the computer monitor up-to-date news stories as well as columns, book and film reviews, and other newspaper features. Some newspapers have a telephone number we can call to listen to portions of the newspaper, such as classified advertisements, before they are printed. Imagine being one of the first to hear about a garage sale and being able to buy things that we don't need before anyone else gets there!

Table 2. Comparison of reading methods

READING METHOD	READING FACTORS		
	Navigation	Comfort	Illustrations
Large print publications	high	high	high
Nonelectronic magnifying devices	low	low	high
CCTV reading	high	medium	high
Computer screen enlargement programs	medium	medium	low
Tape recordings	low	high	low
Speech synthesizers	medium	high	low
Braille on paper	high	high	medium
Braille in electronic form	medium	medium	low

In some geographic areas, we can listen to radio reading services on a special radio receiver. These services read portions or all of the text of local newspapers, including advertising of local merchants. Books, magazines, and other publications may also be read by radio reading services.

Signing our name to checks and other papers

Filling out a check and signing it is easier if we know where to write the date, the amount of the check, and the payee name. A template with holes for filling in this information is helpful. Templates can also be made for other forms that we need to complete on a regular basis.

Taking and leaving messages

A tape recorder can be used to take, send, and receive messages for ourselves or for others. We can leave or receive a message on a tape recorder we share with another person, either blind or sighted. We can make notes for ourselves on a tape recorder; for example, taking notes over the telephone. Tape recorders not much larger than a pack of cigarettes can be used for these purposes.

Organizing a personal collection of information

We have discussed ways of organizing clothes so that we can select matched outfits. We have described a database management program for organizing a collection of magazine articles on leisure activities for visually disabled persons. Now we will look at ways of organizing a personal collection of information.

The information that we wish to organize for easy retrieval is a list of names of individuals and organizations we want to call or write to. This information storage and retrieval system can be relatively simple. We can use a card for each person and each organization and write on each card the name, address, and phone number. The cards would then be filed alphabetically by name of person or organization. Cards for new names would be interfiled. Searching the file would be a matter of looking in the file by name.

This system can also be kept on computer, using either a word processing or a database management program. New names can be added to the list by keying in the appropriate information. The file is searched by name, just like the file on cards. The computer-based file has several advantages over the card file. The program can be used to arrange the names alphabetically when we first prepare the file and when we interfile new names. Searches for names can be made with a search key that will move the cursor to the wanted name. Portions of the file or the entire file can be printed out as mailing labels. This is not to suggest that we buy a computer for this purpose only, but that we may find this as a possible application of a computer we have.

Another example of an information storage and retrieval system is a collection of magazine articles on leisure activities for visually disabled persons, the system used to illustrate a database management program in chapter 2. Here again a manual file or a computer-based file can be used. For a manual file, we might list the names of the hobbies as filing points for the articles; for example, golf, hiking, and swimming. We would then physically file the magazine articles in file folders, each of which would be labelled with the name of the hobby described. If a magazine article is on more than one hobby, we would file the article under one hobby and insert a card with the identification of the magazine article and its filing point in the folder or folders for the other applicable hobbies. Thus, if an article is on both hiking and skiing, we would file it under "Hiking" and insert a card under "Skiing," indicating that an additional article on skiing is filed under "Hiking." An alternative to adding a card in the file folder is to keep a separate card file. Each card would have the name of a hobby as a heading and the identification of the magazine articles that describe this hobby. The cards would be filed alphabetically by hobby. To add new magazine articles to the system, we would insert the new article into an existing folder for a hobby or make a new folder for a hobby described for the first time. Searching the file is a matter of determining under which hobby to look and then selecting the magazine articles from the hobby folder or folders.

The database management program for magazine articles on leisure activities for visually disabled persons described in chapter 2 provides more access points and, therefore, more ways to search the magazine articles. In addition to name of leisure activity, access is provided in six other ways: accession number, bibliographic citation, mental effort entailed, physical effort entailed, needed adaptation for visually disabled persons, and cost. With a database management system, the magazine articles are filed by accession number. The computer record for each magazine article consists of the seven ways of searching the system, listed on a template. Searches are made by calling for a blank template and filling in the search terms under as many headings as are required. The computer then displays completed templates or specified information from the template, such as the accession number, for each magazine article that meets the search specifications. The magazine articles selected in the computer search are then looked up under their accession numbers.

A database management program should be considered for organizing a collection of information or publications if multiple access points per item are required and if searches with a combination of search terms are anticipated. The advantages of computer-based systems over manual files are easier input, searching for a combination of access points, sorting, and printing search output.

Locating cassettes and passages of text on cassette

Let us look at a collection of magazine articles recorded on cassettes. The subject of the article will be the filing point of the cassette. We have identified a specific cassette and are ready to read it by listening to it. We do not want to read the entire article, only one section that discusses the results of a particular study. How can we get to this section of the article on the tape? We can read the tape from the beginning until we get to the part we want. This is not necessary if the tape has been audibly indexed at the beginning of each segment of text. There are two methods for doing this—tone indexing and voice indexing.

Tone indexing

Tone indexing is inserting a sound or beep at certain places on the tape. This may be at the beginning of a chapter or a section of a book or the beginning of the introduction, description of procedure, discussion of results, conclusion, or other portion of a magazine article. To do this, we need a tape recorder with a tone indexing feature. The previously mentioned APH Handi-Cassette tape recorder is one such recorder. We insert a tone on the portion of tape that will be played a few seconds before the passage of text to be marked. The tone is inserted by depressing the play and record buttons and holding the tone index button for a few seconds. The inserted tone is heard when the tape is played at fast forward or on rewind. These audible tones are best inserted at the time the text is recorded. Different meanings might be assigned to tones of different lengths, i.e., a long tone for the beginning of a section and a short tone for the beginning of a chapter.

Voice indexing

While tone indexing is useful for getting quickly to the beginning of a segment of text, such as a chapter in a book, it does not permit access to the contents of a tape by author, subject, or other desired type of access point. Voice indexing permits us to "mark with spoken words" segments of tape. The access points are spoken words that can be heard when the tape is played at fast forward. We will explain the procedure by first describing how a voice-indexed cassette is searched and then how a voice-indexed tape is prepared. To do both of these tasks, we need two tape recorders. One is a standard, commercial tape recorder that plays at standard speed. The second tape recorder is one that needs to be capable of recording on two tracks on each of the two sides of the cassette and to record at fast forward. The previously described APH tape recorder has these features.

Searching a voice-indexed tape. Let us now search a hypothetical voice-indexed cassette. The cassette has recordings of classical jazz played by the bands of Benny Goodman, Louis Armstrong, Duke Ellington, and Count Basie. These selections are recorded on track one of side one. On track two of side one are recorded, at fast forward, the names of the band leaders. The names are recorded so that the musical selection on the parallel track begins just after the corresponding name of the band leader is pronounced.

Here is how we would use this voice indexed tape if we wanted to get to the selection by Count Basie without listening to all of the selections that come before the one we want to hear. We set the APH tape recorder to track two and play it at fast forward until we hear the words "Count Basie." We stop the tape recorder and set it to track one. This should place the tape at or near the beginning of the Count Basie selection. Finding a segment of voice-indexed tape by listening for words played at fast forward takes considerably less time than listening to the tape at regular speed.

Preparation of a voice-indexed cassette. Let us now look at how the words are inserted for voice indexing. We will use the same example of the classical jazz with the same words, the names of the band leaders, used as access points.

We want to record the jazz selections on track one and the names of the band leaders on the parallel track, track two. The names of the band leaders are recorded at fast forward, and the recording of the end of the name is to be followed by the beginning of the corresponding musical selection. We need a recording of the musical selections, a blank cassette, a commercial tape recorder, and an APH tape recorder or another recorder with the aforementioned features. We insert the blank tape into the APH recorder, set it to track two, and record the words "Benny Goodman" on fast forward. We stop the recorder. Then we set the APH recorder to track one and record at regular speed the corresponding musical selection played on our second tape recorder. To voice index and record the second selection, we set the APH recorder to track two, record the words "Louis Armstrong" on fast forward, and stop the recorder. Then we set the APH recorder to track one and record the corresponding musical selection at regular speed. This process of recording the voice indexed words on track two and at fast forward, stopping the recorder, then recording the corresponding musical selection on track one at regular speed is repeated until all of the musical selections have been recorded. Any segment of music or spoken words on cassette can be indexed in this way. Voice indexing was developed by the late Jim Chandler, a sighted librarian who spent much of his retirement time working with blind persons.

Concluding remarks

All of us are seekers, gatherers, consumers, and providers of information. All of us have a PIM to help us with our information-handling activities. Because it generally takes us longer to collect information and read it than it takes sighted persons, it is important for us to be as efficient as possible in our information-handling activities. Hence the emphasis on personal information sources, library search techniques, reading strategy, method of reading, and organization of information.

References

Frank, Mildred. *Seeing with the Brain*, rev. ed. Indianapolis: Council of Citizens with Low Vision International, 1991.

Lauer, Harvey. "Why One Medium Isn't Enough." *OCLC Micro* 5 (December 1989):22-25.

Resources

American Printing House for the Blind
1839 Frankfort Avenue
P.O. Box 6085
Louisville, KY 40206
1-800-223-1839

Associated Services for the Blind Recorded Periodicals
919 Walnut Street
Philadelphia, PA 19107
(215) 627-0600, ext. 208
   Periodicals on anthropology and archeology, computers, business, medicine, science, and ham radio.

National Library Service for the Blind and Physically
 Handicapped (NLS)
1291 Taylor Street NW
Washington, DC 20542
   Call 1-800-424-8567 for the address and phone number of an NLS network library in your area.

Recording for the Blind (RFB)
20 Roszel Road
Princeton, NJ 08540
   Call 1-800-452-0606 for registration information.

4. Jobs for visually disabled persons

Most of us will agree that having a job is a good thing. It may not be a good thing all of the time; every job has its lesser moments. However, the benefits of working far outweigh any disadvantages of most jobs. A job gives us something useful to do, keeps us in touch with the outside world, and enables us to earn a living. If it is a job that we really like, one that we look forward to going to even on a Monday morning, then we are really fortunate. We have different perceptions of what such a job would be because we differ from each other in likes, dislikes, and expectations.

Today blind persons have a greater variety of jobs to choose from than ever before. This is so because of three developments. One is that we live in a more enlightened and benign society than ever before in terms of attitudes toward disabled persons. The change is best illustrated by the passage of civil rights legislation for the disabled in the 1970s and, more recently, by the passage of the Americans with Disabilities Act (ADA) of 1990. ADA makes job discrimination against disabled persons illegal in all but very small organizations and calls for reasonable accommodations to open up employment opportunities for disabled persons.

The second development is the change from an industrial to a postindustrial or information-based society. More and more jobs in business, industry, government, and academe entail the selection, manipulation, retrieval, interpretation, and dissemination of information stored in a computer or accessible at a computer. The third development is the computer and telecommunication technology that makes these new information processing jobs doable by blind persons. Adaptive equipment, such as speech synthesizers, makes it possible for blind persons to use computers on a competitive basis with sighted persons.

Jobs held by blind persons

A rehabilitation counselor recently told me that, when he is asked what jobs blind persons can do, he answers that it would take him considerably less time to list jobs that blind persons can*not* do. Blind persons cannot drive trucks or other vehicles or walk around delivering mail. But such workers are backed up by dispatchers and others in jobs that blind persons can do. The rehabilitation counselor has an impressive list of jobs that blind persons have held or are now holding. Blind persons are or have been medical doctors, congressmen, judges, lawyers, professors, and newspaper reporters. Not every blind person—for that matter, not every sighted person—is capable of performing such jobs. The point is that blind persons with the requisite abilities and perseverance should make the most of what they have and aspire to whatever jobs appeal to them. A partial listing of other jobs held by blind persons, compiled by Job Opportunities for the Blind (JOB), follows in table 3.

Table 3. Selected list of jobs held by blind persons

Computer programmer	Personnel interviewer
Cosmetologist	Quality control specialist
Dispatcher	Rehabilitation counselor
Electrical engineer	Retail sales person
Equal employment officer	Safety engineer
Estate analyst	Social worker
Fundraiser	Teacher of various subjects
Handicapped services coordinator	Telephone sales
Labor relations specialist	Telephone service
Masseur or masseuse	representative for
Medical administrator	Internal Revenue Service
Micrographic technician	Travel agent
Nutrition education coordinator	Volunteer services
Occupational health and safety	coordinator
specialist	Word processor

Not all blind persons work for others. Some own and operate their own businesses, such as mail-order houses, restaurants, and rental agencies.

Preparing oneself to enter or reenter the job market

This section is primarily intended for visually disabled students preparing themselves for a career or jobholders who need to change jobs because of their visual disability. Persons working at a job they can continue to do might be wise to keep that job, even if it has to be modified or performed with the aid of adaptive equipment or with changes in the workplace. Beginning a new career after a number of years in the workforce may put us at a disadvantage, partly because we are in direct competition with younger persons who are just entering the work force and partly because we may not be able to use the experience we gained on the previous job.

Getting a job takes time and effort. In the initial or planning stages, we need to take a hard look at ourselves as a potential employee or business person. This self-examination is intended to tell us what we like to do as well as what we do not like to do and what we are capable of doing or learning as well as what we are not capable of doing or learning. The answers to the questions listed below and the discussion of the answers with a vocational guidance counselor will help us identify our career goals.

- Are we willing to spend four years in college and additional years in a professional school to pursue a career?
- Are we willing to pursue a particular career goal even if experts in the field discourage us from doing so?
- Are we willing to work long hours during the week and on weekends?
- Do we prefer to work with others or by ourselves?
- Do we enjoy helping others?
- Are we willing to keep up with continuing changes in our field?
- Do we prefer to have our job exactly spelled out for us?
- Do we enjoy problem solving?
- How comfortable are we with ambiguous situations?
- How willing are we to take risks?
- How important is making money in our scheme of things?

With the answers to these questions, as well as various tests of skills and aptitudes, our vocational guidance counselor can help us select a career.

The rehabilitation process

We are accustomed to seeking advice from professionals: for medical advice we see a medical doctor; for legal advice we see a lawyer. The professional to see for advice on planning a career is a vocational guidance counselor, specifically one who works with blind persons. These professionals keep up with the job market for blind persons, know training requirements for various jobs, maintain contact with employers, and have knowledge of tests that help in career guidance. Vocational guidance counselors can help us if we are legally blind or have a condition that leads to blindness. Counselors and other professionals are available to us through the agency serving the blind in each state. The names of these agencies vary but they usually have the word "blind" in their title, such as Division of Blind Services or Commission for the Blind. The name, address, and phone number of each of the fifty state agencies are given in the NLS listing of national organizations cited in the references at the end of this chapter.

These agencies are funded by both federal and state funds, and they do much more than offer vocational counseling. What follows is a generic description of the services that we are likely to obtain from the state agency serving the blind. The primary goals of each of these agencies are the same: to help blind persons of all ages to become more independent and to help blind persons of working age to get and keep jobs.

The initial contact with the agency serving the blind is probably by phone. A phone call to the agency will get us an appointment with the vocational guidance counselor, either at the agency's office or at our home. The counselor's job is to match our job potential with a job that makes the most of it. The answers to the questions about careers that we asked ourselves are part of the information that the counselor will use to help us find a job. Additional information will come from tests that we will be asked to take, which may include medical, psychological, social, cultural, vocational, and educational tests. The counselor will use the results of these tests and our discussions to prepare a plan called the Individualized Written Rehabilitation Plan or IWRP. The plan is prepared jointly by the counselor and the client. The IWRP includes a long-range employment goal, intermediate objectives related to the long-range goal, identification of specific rehabilitation services needed, dates of initiation and length of services, and procedure for and schedule of evaluation of the plan. As mentioned before, the plan is intended to provide us with the needed skills for a job that makes the most of our potential.

Learning the needed skills

In addition to and prior to learning job skills, we need to learn independent living skills, mobility skills, and communication skills. Chapter 1 mentioned some of the independent living skills and mobility skills that we need to learn. Communication skills were discussed in chapter 3. These skills are taught by trained rehabilitation teachers. We may be asked to stay in residence during the three to nine months that it takes to learn these skills, or we might go to a rehabilitation center on a daily basis, just as we would go to a job. In some cases, the rehabilitation teacher may work with us at home. Perhaps the most important result of this rehabilitation is the renewed confidence that we will have gained in ourselves. We will have learned that by being able to perform these different tasks, we will be ready to resume a normal life. That includes getting the needed education and training for a job and competing with sighted persons for jobs. Getting ready for a job may entail going to a college, university, or trade school. Instead of or in addition to formal training, we may have on-the-job training.

A few words should be said about who pays for all of this training. The agency for the blind is authorized to pay for rehabilitation training as well as training for jobs. It may also pay for costs associated with such training, such as daily living expenses, transportation costs, medical expenses, cost of adaptive equipment, tuition for course work, textbooks, and readers. While the agency is authorized to pay for expenses associated with training blind persons, it may or may not have funds to pay for all of these expenses. Organizations for the blind have scholarship funds for students, as do foundations and other private organizations. Directories of organizations that have programs of financial assistance are kept in libraries.

Finding a job

All of this studying and training is intended to lead to one thing: a job that we like. How do we go about getting such a job? The vocational guidance counselor can offer incentives to potential employers, including tax breaks for hiring disabled persons and payment by the agency of part or all of our salary during a trial period. The counselor can discuss with the employer the need, if any, for job modification, changes in the workplace, or the use of adaptive equipment such as computer output via speech synthesizers.

We use the good offices of the vocational guidance counselor but also do some job hunting on our own. We can get a listing on cassette of jobs for blind persons from the previously mentioned Job Opportunities for the Blind. JOB is a joint project of the National Federation of the Blind and the U.S. Department of Labor. It is free to blind job seekers and provides various services, including job listings and workshops. The 1991 JOB seminar included talks about job interviews, jobs in newspapers and radio, and jobs for free-lance writers.

Three other publications about jobs should be mentioned. In *Career Perspectives: Interviews with Blind and Visually Impaired Persons* (see references), five professionals tell us how they got where they are and what helped them get there. The workers interviewed include a research scientist, an urban planner, a personnel analyst, an assistant U.S. attorney, and a clinical psychologist.

The Hadley School for the Blind (see references) offers a noncredit course on careers in computers. It consists of interviews with blind persons who make use of computers in their jobs. The jobs range from word processing to computer system management. Each interviewee talks about the job, what the training requirements are, and what personal characteristics are required for the job.

A list of high-tech jobs held by visually disabled persons is maintained by the American Foundation for the Blind's Career and Technology Information Bank (see references). More than 1,200 visually disabled persons are included in the listing. We can get names and addresses of persons on the list. The spring 1992 issue of *Dialogue* (see references) has several articles about jobs for the blind.

Two other skills are needed when we look for a job. We need to be able to prepare a good résumé and we need to be good at interviewing employers. The idea is to make the best possible impression in the résumé and the interview. The résumé, or short biographical sketch, need not be longer than a typewritten page. It should give facts about us—name, address, phone number, education, and jobs held, if any. We might want to include our hobbies and outside activities to give employers a better view of us. This is a general-purpose résumé, prepared in multiple copies and sent to potential employers with a cover letter. In the cover letter we address the specific job and give reasons why we think we are better than anybody else for the job.

Both the cover letter and the interview require more information. We want to find out about the employer and about the job ahead of time, if possible. Again, descriptions of employing organizations can be found in directories in the public library.

Interviewing employers requires skills in answering as well as asking questions. At the risk of being redundant, let me restate that we are trying to make the best impression possible and to convince the employer that we are the best person for the job. Here are a few hints to consider for the interview:

- Dress neatly for the occasion.
- Get there on time.
- Show enthusiasm.
- Be prepared to answer all types of questions about yourself.
- Be prepared to ask questions about the job.
- Be prepared to answer the question, "Why should you be given the job?"

Our first interview may not result in a job offer. We will, however, have learned from that experience and will do better next time. Résumé writing and interviewing skills are discussed at meetings of organizations for the blind. A cassette tape of a talk on job interviews presented at the 1991 meeting of the American Federation for the Blind is available free from JOB.

References

Blindness and Visual Impairments: National Information and Advocacy Organizations. Reference Circular 90-2. Washington, DC: National Library Service for the Blind and Physically Handicapped, December 1992.

Career Perspectives: Interviews with Blind and Physically Impaired Professionals. New York: American Foundation for the Blind, 1990.

Dialogue. Spring 1992.
   This issue includes several articles on jobs held by visually disabled persons. A copy of this issue may be borrowed from the NLS network library.

Hadley School for the Blind. Careers in computers.
   A noncredit course on cassette available from
Hadley School for the Blind
700 Elm Street
Winnetka, IL 60093
1-800-323-4238

Resources

American Foundation for the Blind
Career and Technology Information Bank
15 West 16th Street
New York, NY 10011
1-800-232-5463

Job Opportunities for the Blind (JOB)
1800 Johnson Street
Baltimore, MD 21230
1-800-638-7518
   Provides free cassette listings of jobs, workshops on interviewing, and other job-related topics.

5. *Leisure activities for visually disabled persons*

How would we spend our time if we could do anything that we wanted to do? Of course, all of us are under constraints, be they visual, financial, or other; but all of us do, or should, have time that we can call our own and with which we can do whatever we like. This is our leisure or recreation time, and ways of spending it are suggested in this chapter.

We have a wide variety of activities from which to choose. For the purpose of convenience, the activities are placed in three groups: activities that provide primarily mental exercise, activities that provide primarily physical exercise, and activities that we do as volunteers to help others.

Within these groupings, activities can be further differentiated by where they are done, with how many others, and at what financial cost. Some activities can be done at home, some can be done only away from home, and some either at home or away from home. There are outdoor and indoor activities, activities that cost nothing, and those that cost a lot. References to literature on hobbies are given at the end of the chapter. In many cases, clubs or organizations interested in a particular hobby can supply information about it. Local as well as national hobby groups can be identified with the help of directories and special files kept by the public library.

Mental activities

We can choose from different levels of mental activities, ranging from those that do not present a challenge to those that take all the thinking that we can muster. Sometimes the same activity can be approached at different levels, for example, chess or reading. Two activities, reading and shortwave radio listening, are discussed in some detail as examples of activities with common elements. Both cost very little to pursue. Both are typically done by oneself, although the experience can be shared with others. Both can be done at home or away from home, and both can be done either indoors or outdoors.

Reading

We will assume that either large-print books or books on cassette are needed for our recreational reading. Books in either of these two formats can be borrowed from the public library.

There is also a library service especially designed for us: the National Library Service for the Blind and Physically Handicapped (NLS). NLS provides us with a wide choice of recorded and brailled material, along with playback equipment and book lists to help us with our reading selection. We will restrict our discussion to recorded material, except to say that NLS provides books, magazines, and lists of books in braille. All of this library service is delivered to our home at no cost to us. We are eligible for the service if we cannot read or handle print materials because of visual or physical disabilities. Legal blindness is not an eligibility requirement. NLS service is obtained through one of the 146 network libraries. To register for the service we complete an application form obtained from the NLS network library that serves our area. The local public library will know the location of this network library and may have copies of the application form. A professional in the field of eye care or a librarian can certify our eligibility for the service. The completed application is sent to the local network library.

Books and magazines to be recorded by NLS are selected with input from network librarians and users of the service. The recorded books are sent to network libraries for circulation to their users. Individual issues of recorded magazines on flexible discs are mailed directly to subscribers by the producers of the discs.

As NLS users, we may borrow playback equipment, cassette machines, and disc players for as long as we use the service. Neither cassettes nor discs are played at commercial speed and cannot, therefore, be played on commercial equipment unless it is designed for playing NLS recordings. Cassettes are played at half the commercial speed and on four tracks per cassette. Discs are played at one-fourth the speed of long-playing records. The tape and disc machines are mailed to our home and are returned postage-free to the network library if they need to be repaired. Repairs are made at no cost to us. Earphones can be used with this equipment for privacy, to avoid disturbing others, or for special hearing needs.

Magazines from NLS

We can subscribe to one or more of the forty-three magazines recorded by NLS on flexible discs. Recorded magazines include *The Atlantic*, *Sports Illustrated*, and *U.S. News and World Report*. Monthly issues of *The Atlantic* on flexible discs, for example, arrive at our home within a month of the arrival of print copies at newsstands. The entire text of the print edition is included, except for advertisements, illustrations, and puzzles. Each disc takes about one hour per side to read at normal reading speed; thus, the typical issue of *The Atlantic*, recorded on seven sides, takes about seven hours to read from end to end at normal reading speed. The disc player has variable speed control so we can play discs at speeds either faster or slower than the normal reading rate.

Books from NLS

We can choose from more than 60,000 recorded books in the NLS collection—detective stories, science fiction, best-selling novels, biographies, current events, poetry, and the classics of literature and history. There are books for every taste. Books for children and books in foreign languages are also found in the collection but not in great numbers. NLS records the full text of each book. It does not record the illustrations, the index, and, for some books, the list of references. The NLS cassette machine has variable speed controls so that we can either speed up or slow down the recording. At normal reading speed, it takes six hours to listen to the four tracks of one NLS cassette. Typically, a book of fiction is recorded on two cassettes and takes seven to twelve hours to read.

As part of the service, we receive a bimonthly publication called *Taking Book Topics*, which gives a brief description of newly recorded books available from the NLS network libraries. *Talking Book Topics* comes to us in either large-print or flexible disc format. We can select newly recorded books from this publication on the basis of information given for each book, including title, author, narrator, length, format (cassette or flexible disc), language (English or foreign), level (adult or child), presence or absence of strong language, violence, or descriptions of sex.

To order books listed in an issue of *Talking Book Topics*, we can complete the order form in the publication and send it to our network library, or we can call the library. The network library can also be telephoned to request any book in the NLS collection. If we live near the network library, we can also visit the library and select our reading material there.

The books are delivered by mail. To return a book, postage-free, we reverse the address label on the book container so that the network library address shows and send it back.

We can read NLS talking books and magazines on discs anywhere there is an electric outlet. We can read NLS talking books on cassette indoors or outdoors, since the cassette machine has a rechargeable battery that plays for about eight hours.

Whether we have a few minutes or a few hours, reading is a most pleasant way of spending our leisure time. The selection of reading material provided by NLS ranges from escape novels that require mostly suspension of disbelief and little mental effort to intellectually challenging books on science, philosophy, and many other fascinating topics.

Shortwave radio listening

Shortwave radio listening gives us an ear to the world. We can hear news from London, Paris, Tokyo, Moscow, and other world capitals. Overseas stations usually broadcast to us in English. Their news broadcasts are not only about what is happening in their countries but also about what is happening in our country, seen from a different perspective. A case in point is Alistair Cooke's "Letter from America," an insightful and wry commentary broadcast weekly on the British Broadcasting Corporation (BBC). It is equally interesting to hear what the Voice of America, our government's shortwave radio station, is saying about us to people in different parts of the world.

Each country has its own musical signature for identification. When we hear "Yankee Doodle Dandy," we know that we are listening to the Voice of America. When we hear the chimes of Big Ben, we are listening to the BBC. The BBC has frequent news broadcasts, often followed by a review of the British press, during which excerpts or British newspaper editorials are read. The BBC also broadcasts plays, short stories, quiz shows, interviews, and book reviews, and all of this without commercials.

The sound of the "Blue Danube Waltz" tells us that we are listening to Radio Austria. In addition to news about Austria, we can hear concerts of Austrian folk music and descriptions of charming Austrian alpine villages that sound so picturesque we want to visit them. Radio Moscow, formerly identified by the martial sounds of "The Internationale," the Communist anthem, offers a variety of interesting programs about Russia, its people, art, and culture. One program, "Moscow Mailbag," answers listeners' questions about Russia, giving us insights about the land, its people, and its culture.

News, documentaries, interviews, concerts, and language lessons are some of the types of programs that we can listen to on shortwave radio.

Shortwave radio receivers can be bought for as little as $50 but can cost over $1,000. All shortwave radios will enable us to listen to broadcasts from overseas without an outside antenna. We might want to start with an inexpensive set and buy more expensive equipment later. More expensive receivers and an outside antenna will give a wider choice of stations and better sound quality.

Typically, shortwave reception is better out in the open. Reception varies with atmospheric conditions and time of day; usually, it is better in the evening. Once we have bought our shortwave receiver, our only listening expense is the cost of house current or batteries.

A shortwave radio is for listening only. If we wish to send messages to others, we are dealing with a different hobby, amateur or ham radio. To be a ham radio operator, one must pass a test and obtain a license. One also must buy the needed broadcasting and receiving equipment. Courses in ham radio operation are offered free by the Hadley School for the Blind.

Writing

Writing can be a very satisfying hobby. We might write an article for the newsletter of a local organization. We may want to share the history of our family with other family members. We might try creative writing—poetry, short stories, or novels.

We will probably not get rich from the sale of our writing. Publications such as *Dialogue* pay only token amounts for contributions. But even if our writing reaches only a small audience, we will have the pleasure of pursuing a hobby. There is satisfaction in putting our thoughts on paper or a computer screen, in outlining, writing, and rewriting, and then seeing the final product.

Writing to family and friends is another way of sharing our thoughts. Magazines for the blind, such as *Dialogue* and *Mathilda Ziegler Magazine for the Blind*, list pen pals with special interests whom we can contact. If we write in large print, in braille, or in recorded form, we can send our correspondence postage-free.

Enrolling in courses

One way to learn creative writing is to enroll in a course. We might consider enrolling in an adult education course on this or another subject. Courses that are free or cost little are offered by adult education agencies in most communities. The Hadley School for the Blind offers free correspondence courses on a variety of subjects. The courses are on cassettes or in braille and high school credit is offered, if desired.

Here is another possibility: we can learn to play a musical instrument at home and without cost for the instruction. NLS offers instruction on cassette for learning to play the piano, organ, harmonica, guitar, banjo, recorder, and accordion.

Attending cultural events

Going to museums or the theater is usually a pleasant outing. Some museums rent or lend without charge audiotapes that describe the exhibits; some theaters supply blind persons with audiotapes that describe visual cues in the performance.

Card and board games

Board games with enlarged characters or illustrations or braille markings are for sale by mail-order houses that specialize in products for the blind. Also available are playing cards with either large-print or braille markings. For those of us who are dedicated bridge or poker players, this might be an inducement to learn braille symbols for letters and numbers.

Computers for fun and games

Computers can be used for fun as well as for work. Computer games can be bought as software packages or are available on commercial information services such as Prodigy (discussed in chapter 2). Many of these games require some usable sight. We might want to ask about sight requirements before we buy software.

Learning a computer language for the fun of it is another possible hobby that will give us mental exercise. One note of warning—programming may become addictive and take up all of our time.

Physical activities

Physical exercise is good for the body and the soul. A long walk, a bike ride, or another form of exercise is likely to relax us both physically and mentally and give us a generally better perspective. Nothing says that poor eyesight should exclude us from physical exercise. Walking is one form of exercise that we can do either alone or with a sighted companion. We can bike if we ride on a tandem bicycle with a sighted companion in front.

Tandem riding

I hope that I will be forgiven if I draw on personal experience to discuss tandem riding. Biking was one of the pleasures that I thought I would have to give up with loss of my sight. I thought that until one day my wife came to pick me up after work. Instead of sitting behind the wheel of our car, she sat on the front seat of a tandem bicycle that I had never seen before. It was new to me but not to the world, a Schwinn, vintage World

War II, with balloon tires, coaster brakes, and only one speed: very slow. The two sets of handlebars did not match and the metal frame was rusty. I must confess that I was a bit reluctant to get on the back seat, partly because of the bike's appearance and partly because I had not biked for a number of years. I overcame my reluctance and, with a good deal of huffing and puffing, rode the mile or so from the office to home. Soon we used the bike not only for commuting to work but for rides around the neighborhood and, after a while, for rides of up to twenty miles.

We learned to synchronize our pedalling and I learned that the captain, the person sitting in front, was in command of the vehicle. As stroker, I had to start pedalling when the captain started pedalling and I had to stop pedalling when she did. Soon we outgrew our first tandem and sold it for what we paid for it, about fifty dollars. Our second came from a large mail-order house. It was as heavy as the first one (about seventy pounds) and had matching handlebars and five speeds. By then, we had bought a tandem carrier for the top of the car so that we could take the bike to a good starting point for our bike ride. But the new bike was not built to take the long rides that we wanted to take. After walking instead of riding the tandem to the car for the third time because of a broken spoke, we decided that we needed another tandem, one that could be used for long-distance biking. We sold the second tandem for about $300, roughly what we paid for it, and bought one that weighs only forty-two pounds, has fifteen speeds, and does not mind going up hills. Although $1,800 seemed a lot to pay for it at the time, we have used it for six years and it is still going strong.

We took the tandem to Europe, where my wife and I on our tandem and a friend on a bicycle built for one pedalled about a thousand miles in six weeks. We took helmets, bicycle pumps, and about ten pounds of clothing per person stored in paniers. We arrived in Luxembourg on a morning in June. It was raining and about forty degrees cooler than when we departed from Florida. My wife and our friend had to put the pedals and handlebars back on the bikes and reconnect the brake cables. Then we had to go into town to look for a room at a rate that fit our budget. The rain was still coming down hard and it looked as though it was going to be a very long trip. But we found a cheap hotel and, after a good night's sleep, things started to look better. We enjoyed our first European breakfast and the sun came out. We were able to put our bicycles in the baggage car of the train (we had not been sure whether that would be possible) and took a long train ride to Austria, our first destination. In Austria, we biked along the Danube from the German border to Hungary. Then we took a train to France and biked from Alsace-Lorraine through Belgium into Holland. From there we completed the trip by train into Luxembourg.

Meeting and talking with people in the small towns that we passed through were some of the most pleasant experiences of the trip. It was easy to meet people. They had not seen many Americans who were no longer in their prime and on bicycles. We avoided big cities and busy highways because of the traffic. We did get lost several times. After some practice, we worked out a way of asking for directions. Since I speak French and German, I was appointed spokesman. My female companions pointed me to face the person that I was addressing, and they were in charge of seeing and interpreting the hand signals given to us. We also used a small tape recorder to record the directions so that we could listen to them at appropriate intervals. Most of the time this worked fine. When it did not, we found alternate places to go to and enjoy. And there was a lot to enjoy—the people, the food and drink, the sounds and smells of the villages and the countryside. Tandem riding has given us the opportunity to meet many people, both in Europe and in the United States, where we belong to a tandem club. It is also very good exercise.

Other sports

We can enjoy other sports and physical activities. Some sports need to be modified to compensate for our visual disability. The modification may be made by adding sound to the equipment used in the sport or by using a sighted companion. Balls with a beeping sound are used by blind persons to play baseball and basketball. In these two sports the bases and the net also emit sounds. Sports we can pursue with the assistance of a sighted companion include golf, mountain climbing, snow skiing, and running.

Other physical activities to choose from (some of which are described in publications listed at the end of the chapter) include boating, canoeing, camping, fishing, gardening, square dancing, and swimming.

Volunteer activities

There is a saying that it is more blessed to give than to receive. As visually disabled persons we tend to be more on the receiving end of volunteer efforts. Nothing is wrong with this; no matter how independent we are, we do need help from sighted persons. But we can also help others, give some time to the community in which we live, and feel good about ourselves. Fringe benefits of volunteering are meeting new people and opening ourselves to new experiences. Working as volunteers gives us a means of interacting with the sighted world. We can also learn new skills as volunteers, some of which might be useful on the job. What we can do as volunteers will depend on what skills we have, what new skills we are willing and able to learn, the extent of our visual disability, where we are able to do the work, and how much time we have for it. There is another selection criterion that is important: we should enjoy the volunteer work and get something out of it.

Teaching

One example of a volunteer project to consider is teaching English as a second language. Refugees from Asia, Latin America, and other parts of the world have a language handicap when they come to this country. They can see print and hear conversation but they cannot understand English. We can help them learn. After a dozen or so hours of instruction in a course on how to tutor, offered by a community agency, we are ready to work with our first foreign student. We do not need to read print for this instruction. Our student wants to learn English for coping with everyday tasks, such as shopping or asking for directions. We simulate these tasks by asking and answering questions and thus teach English words and grammar. After the students increase their English vocabulary, we can ask them to read a newspaper and discuss its contents with us. Chances are that we will not only enlarge the students' vocabulary and teach them about our country but also learn about their country and culture. Seeing our students' proficiency in English improve on a weekly basis can be very satisfying.

Mediating

Another volunteer activity that I enjoy is being a mediator in small claims court. Cases in small claims courts, like those in other courts, are subject to delays because of the caseload. Our judicial system allows anybody to sue anybody else for any reason. Many people do so. In small claims court in Florida, which takes suits for up to $2,500, neither the plaintiff nor the defendant may use a lawyer. To reduce the backlog of cases and to reduce court expenses, mediators are used. Mediators are court-trained and court-appointed volunteers who are assigned to hear cases before they go on trial. Often the mediator can resolve the dispute between plaintiff and defendant and thus reduce the number of cases a judge must hear.

My wife had mediated for about three years when she suggested that I try this as a volunteer activity. I had my doubts, but because my wife had come up with good ideas in the past (even though they did not sound good at first), I decided to give it a try. I enrolled in the formal training program of about twenty hours, observed mediators, and was observed, in turn, before I became a certified mediator.

The mediation procedure goes something like this. When a case is assigned to a mediator, he or she picks up the case folder and walks with the plaintiff and the defendant to a hearing room. The three sit around a table and the mediator explains the objectives of mediation and the procedure, and tries to get the opposing parties to talk to each other and agree on a way to settle their dispute. If an agreement is reached, the mediator writes it up as a conditional judgment, a contract that both parties and the mediator sign. If the disputing parties cannot come to an agreement, the case is set for court.

The procedure I used at first as a mediator was to sit in the hearing room and have another mediator bring in the disputing parties along with a folder for the case. The sighted mediator would read the case folder for me. I would then do the mediation and dictate the agreement to the sighted mediator or have the mediator indicate on the contract form that the case should be scheduled for court. I was not satisfied with this arrangement because I had to use another volunteer, the sighted mediator, in order to mediate. I now use the plaintiff to read and write for me. I walk into the hearing room with the disputing parties and the case folder and, after explaining the objectives and procedures, ask the plaintiff to read the salient facts of the case for me, the names and addresses of plaintiff and defendant, and the amount of money involved. If an agreement can be reached, I dictate the agreement to the plaintiff. The plaintiff reads the agreement back to make sure that it has been properly recorded and is agreed to by the defendant. This procedure has worked so far. If and when I get a case with a plaintiff who cannot read or write, or if other problems occur, I will ask for help, just as other mediators do.

Other volunteer activities

Margaret Smith suggests several other volunteer activities in her book (see references). These include working for political candidates by manning the telephone, stuffing envelopes, or doing other necessary tasks; doing telephone counseling; and telephoning elderly persons on a regular basis. We can find out about volunteer opportunities by contacting agencies that coordinate such activities.

We can choose from among many recreational activities, based on our interests, available time, and available resources. It takes some time to learn the activity and time before we can tell whether or not it is the right one for us. If we find that one activity is not for us, we can always find another one.

References

General magazines on cassette

Choice Magazine for Listening
85 Channel Drive
Port Washington, NY 11050
> Free of charge from publisher.

Dialogue
Blindskills
P.O. Box 5181
Salem, OR 97304

The spring 1992 issue has articles on tandem bicycle riding, golf, creative writing, and gardening. Most issues include articles on hobbies.

Mathilda Ziegler Magazine for the Blind
20 West 17th Street
New York, NY 10011
Free of charge from publisher.

Books, parts of books, or lists of references on recreation

Living with Low Vision: A Resource Guide for People with Sight Loss. Lexington, KY: Resources for Rehabilitation Inc., 1990.

Ludwig, Irene, Lynne Luxton, and Marie Attmore. *Creative Recreation for Blind and Visually Impaired Adults*. New York: American Foundation for the Blind, 1988.

NLS Leisure Pursuits series

The separate booklets in large print, flexible disc, or braille are available on the following topics: bird watching, fishing, horses, sailing, swimming, and skiing. Each booklet in this series includes bibliographies, lists of organizations, and other resources.

Reddington, Robert. *On the Move in the Great Outdoors*. 1992. On cassette for $5 from
Massachusetts Association for the Blind
200 Ivy Street
Brookline, MA 02146
Describes techniques blind people can employ when hiking, camping, tandem bicycle riding, canoeing, rowing, and cross-country skiing.

Rickards, Peter. *Popular Activities and Games for Blind, Visually Impaired and Disabled People*. Brighton Beach, Australia: Association for the Blind, 1986.

Smith, Margaret M. *If Blindness Strikes, Don't Strike Out: A Lively Look at Living with Visual Impairment*. Springfield, IL: Charles C Thomas, 1984. (RC 21060)

Publications about individual recreational activities for blind persons

Astronomy

Grice, Noreen A. "Touching the Sky." *Sky & Telescope* 80 (July 1990):79-82.

Games

Sports, Outdoor Recreation, and Games for Visually and Physically Impaired Individuals. Reference Circular 91-1. Washington, DC: NLS, May 1991.
Lists vendors of checkers, cribbage, and other games in a format usable by visually disabled persons.

Ham radio

QST is a magazine of interest to hobbyists who send as well as receive radio messages. The magazine is available on disc, free of charge, from NLS.

Mountain climbing

Stewart, Doug. "Climbing Blind: Colorado Mountain School Teaches People How to Conquer Their Limitations." *National Parks* 62(May-June 1989):22-26.

Museums

Seligmann, Jean. "Please Touch the Art Works: Seeing Through Feeling." *Newsweek* (November 6, 1989):77.

Shore, Irma, ed. *Access to Art: A Museum Directory for Blind and Visually Impaired People*. New York: American Foundation for the Blind, 1989.

6. The blindness system

We have discussed components of the "blindness system" throughout this book, even though we have not called it that. The blindness system is made up of all visually disabled persons, organizations of visually disabled persons, and organizations charged with providing services for visually disabled persons. Organizations of the blind can be national or local; they can be concerned with all aspects of the lives of visually disabled persons or with specialized aspects. Organizations charged with providing services for the blind include government and private agencies that provide rehabilitation services, advocacy groups, and commercial enterprises that specialize in products for blind persons.

In this chapter, we will provide a closer look at how we can interact with the blindness system and will mention benefits that may be available to us because of our disability.

Independence for visually disabled persons

Before we deal with these topics, a few words are in order about independence for the visually disabled. Complete independence for the visually disabled may be the ultimate objective, but it is one that cannot now be achieved. There are times when we need help from sighted persons, whether it is to read a handwritten note or to find our way in an unfamiliar environment. We are not the only people who need help; everybody needs help at some time or other. Our goal should be to become as independent as possible, with the understanding that there will be circumstances when help will be needed from sighted persons.

Help from sighted persons

Help will come from sighted persons, sometimes upon request, sometimes volunteered, sometimes wanted and needed, sometimes neither wanted nor needed. The last point was illustrated in an educational film used to teach sighted persons how to act in the presence of a blind person. In one of the scenes a sighted person "helped" a blind man to cross the street by carrying him across. The blind man did not want to cross the street. The lesson is that one should ask before being helpful and that there are better ways to help a blind person cross the street than carrying him. Sighted persons we meet are likely to have had little contact with blind persons, to have some misunderstandings about blindness, and to be uncomfortable in our presence. I have met many persons who were surprised to hear that most blind persons have some residual sight and that most do not use braille for reading and writing. Sighted persons are uncomfortable when they first meet a blind person because they do not know how to act. This is our chance to be proactive instead of reactive and to do a little educating at the same time.

Here are a few suggestions for making the sighted person feel at ease in our presence. Tell him or her that it is okay to use words such as "see" or "look" and other words dealing with sight. Conversation becomes awkward without these commonly used words. We might want to tell him how much or little we actually see. If help is needed, we should make clear what help we need. It is also a good idea to overlook what we consider inappropriate responses, probably caused by the person's not knowing what to say or do. We should demonstrate by word and deed that we are no different from any other person, except that we have problems seeing.

Benefits for visual disability

Now for a philosophical question: Should we accept the benefits offered us because of our visual disability? Each of us has answered this question, either explicitly or implicitly. The answer may be based on our financial circumstances and our system of beliefs. We may not have the luxury of being able to refuse the benefits that society has for us. My own answer, for what it is worth, follows. The loss of sight brings with it the need to spend more time, effort, and money on some things than sighted persons do. Two examples will illustrate this point: we read more slowly than most sighted persons and it usually takes us longer to get from place to place than it does sighted persons. I conclude from this that we should accept the benefits government and private organizations offer.

I have discussed in previous chapters the rehabilitation and related services provided by state agencies for the blind. Veterans, whether or not their sight loss is service-connected, can obtain similar services from the Department of Veterans Affairs. I have also discussed library services to which we are entitled because of our disability. Additional benefits are available to us from other sources. The federal government offers several such benefits, some for all legally blind persons and some only for those with another special need. An example of the latter is social security supplemental income for blind persons who earn less than a specified amount per year. The Social Security Administration has a book on cassette that describes programs and benefits (see references). Legally blind taxpayers can claim an additional deduction on their federal income tax. Some localities have reduced real estate taxes for legally blind persons. To qualify for such tax reductions, obtain a statement of legal blindness from an eye specialist and file it with the tax authorities. We can vote by absentee ballot even though we may be in town on election day. This gives us a chance to study the ballot beforehand and helps us avoid any mobility problems at the polls. We may send mail postage free if it is written in large print or braille or is in recorded form.

Public transportation

We are entitled to reduced fares and/or special treatment when we travel by taxi, bus, train, or plane. In many towns, a reduced-cost taxi service, subsidized by federal funds, is available to transport disabled persons to and from work or elsewhere. Tickets for Amtrak trains can be purchased at reduced rates. If we take along a sighted companion, he or she rides free on Greyhound buses. Airlines, although they do not give reduced fares for visually disabled persons, provide special services for us. We need not be apprehensive about flying unaccompanied to a city in this country or in Europe. Airline personnel will, once we have identified ourselves as visually disabled, board us ahead of the other passengers, bring us braille safety instructions (even if we do not read braille), help us deplane, get us to another plane if necessary, help us retrieve our baggage, and get us a taxi. On an unaccompanied plane trip to Europe, an airline employee even went with me to the duty-free store and helped me pick out cigars as presents. As one of my blind friends once remarked, airlines treat us as fragile, perishable, and very expensive freight, and they make sure that we get to where we are going.

Organizations of and for the blind

In chapter 3, we discussed the benefits of attending meetings and conventions of organizations, including organizations of the blind. Attending such meetings and reading the organizations' publications help us keep up with topics of interest to us, such as changes in the job market, in computer equipment, or in legislation affecting blind persons. The NLS publication on national organizations includes a list of organizations of and for the blind. Another NLS publication lists organizations involved in sports and outdoor recreation activities (see references).

Support groups

There may be times when we just want to talk with other persons who also have problems with their eyes—perhaps to share what has helped us or to get a different perspective on a problem. Two or more persons with similar problems can form a support group to discuss them. The term "peer counseling" is sometimes used for such informal discussions. These discussions can be held over the phone or in someone's home or any other convenient place. Agencies that serve the blind may know about support groups in a given area. Such groups are particularly valuable to persons who have recently suffered a sight loss.

So here it is: We want to be as independent as possible, but there are some tasks that we can do only with the assistance of others. Assistance is available not only from individuals but also from organizations that are willing, ready, and able to help, when that is needed.

References

NLS. *Blindness and Visual Impairments: National Information and Advocacy Organizations*. Reference Circular 90-2. Washington, DC: NLS, December 1992.

    Includes names, addresses, telephone numbers, and brief descriptions of private organizations as well as names, addresses, and telephone numbers of agencies in the fifty states responsible for the administration of special education and rehabilitation funds.

NLS. *Sports, Outdoor Recreation, and Games for Visually and Physically Impaired Individuals*. Reference Circular 91-1. Washington, DC: NLS, May 1991.

    Lists names, addresses, and phone numbers of national organizations that sponsor athletic events at various levels and provide related services for children, youth, and adults. A brief description of activities is given for most listings.

Social Security Administration. *Social Security Programs and Benefits*.

    A cassette recording of the agency's pamphlets entitled "Understanding Social Security," "Retirement," "Survivors," "Medicare Coverage," "Disability," and "Supplemental Income" is available from NLS network libraries. (RC 33141)

Index

ISBN 0-16-041749-X

9 780160 417498   90000